Bittersweet Victory

Tales of Respiratory Therapists Working to Save Lives During the COVID-19 Pandemic

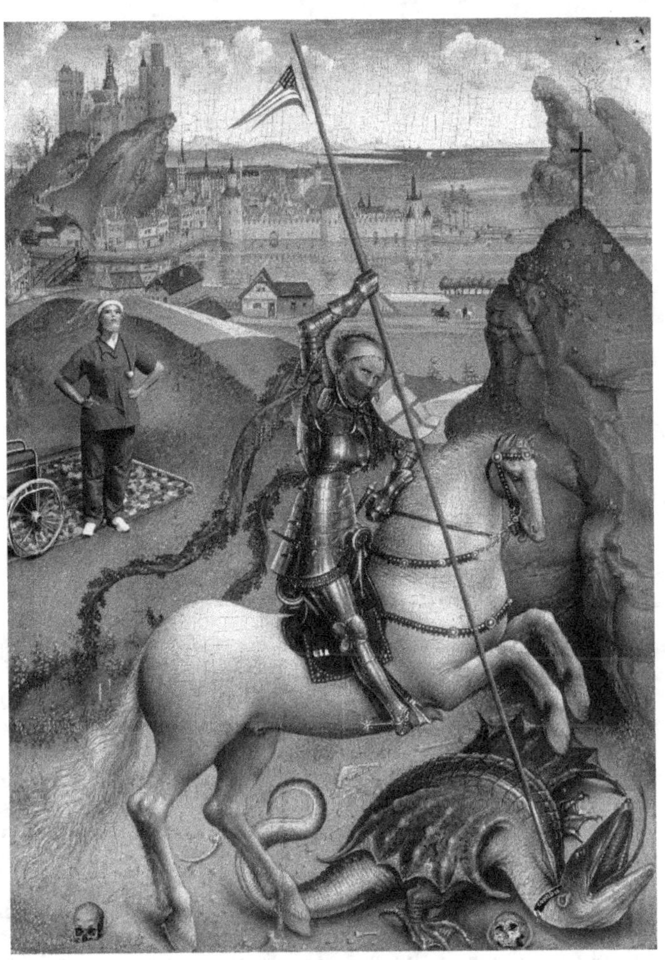

By
Riley O'Neal

Copyright © 2023

Published in the United States of America
by Amazon Kindle Direct Publishing.

Cover artwork design: Riley O'Neal
Interior design: Riley O'Neal, Font: Georgia

All scriptures are taken from the *public domain* World English Bible unless otherwise indicated. All references to Hebrew "Yahweh" have been changed to "God" and "Yah" to "the Lord". Some verses have been modified to reflect current times more accurately and may not be noted on the specific page in this book in order to provide less distraction to the readers. Please refer to the World English Bible for the original translation, if interested.

Most of the artwork is derived from Renaissance paintings that are within the Public Domain of their respective countries of origin, the United States of America, and/or areas where the copyright term is the author's life plus a certain number of years (75 - 100).

ISBN 9798878271165 (paperback) 9798882675317 (hardback)

Printed in the United States of America.

Library of Congress Control Number: 2024903927

Preface

This book is dedicated to my mother, may God rest her soul, a devout and loving Christian and steadfast member of the Church of Christ all her life. And to my beautiful wife, without whom I could not have finished this book.

This book attempts to retell, as accurately as possible, true events experienced by actual *Respiratory Therapists* and other medical professionals who were their allies in the battles on the frontline of the Covid-19 Pandemic.

Respiratory Therapists (RTs) are the medically licensed professionals in the United States of America who have been specifically trained regarding diagnosis and treatment of patients with respiratory diseases, among other things. RTs are the administrators of medicines, medical procedures, and mechanical ventilators to help patients suffering from any/all respiratory diseases. These include, but are not limited to acute Asthma, Bronchitis, Cystic Fibrosis, Emphysema, Pneumonia, Tuberculosis, and Acute Respiratory Distress Syndromes (ARDS) such as Covid-19.

RTs are also responsible for obtaining and interpreting Arterial Blood Gases (ABGs). An ABG is a procedure to draw oxygenated blood from a patient's artery (usually the radial artery in the wrist of the arm).

An ABG can be an extremely painful procedure if a nerve is nicked during the arterial puncture of the patient's arm.

However, most experienced RTs have developed skills to accurately pinpoint the artery and miss any surrounding nerves, thus causing little or no pain to the patient.

RTs cover all areas of a hospital from the Emergency Room (ER) to the Intensive Care Unit (ICU) and all the floors in between!

Disclaimer

All names and places have been changed to protect the privacy of those involved. Any fictional character in the artwork that has a likeness to any person whether living or dead, is purely coincidental.

Contents

Chapter One

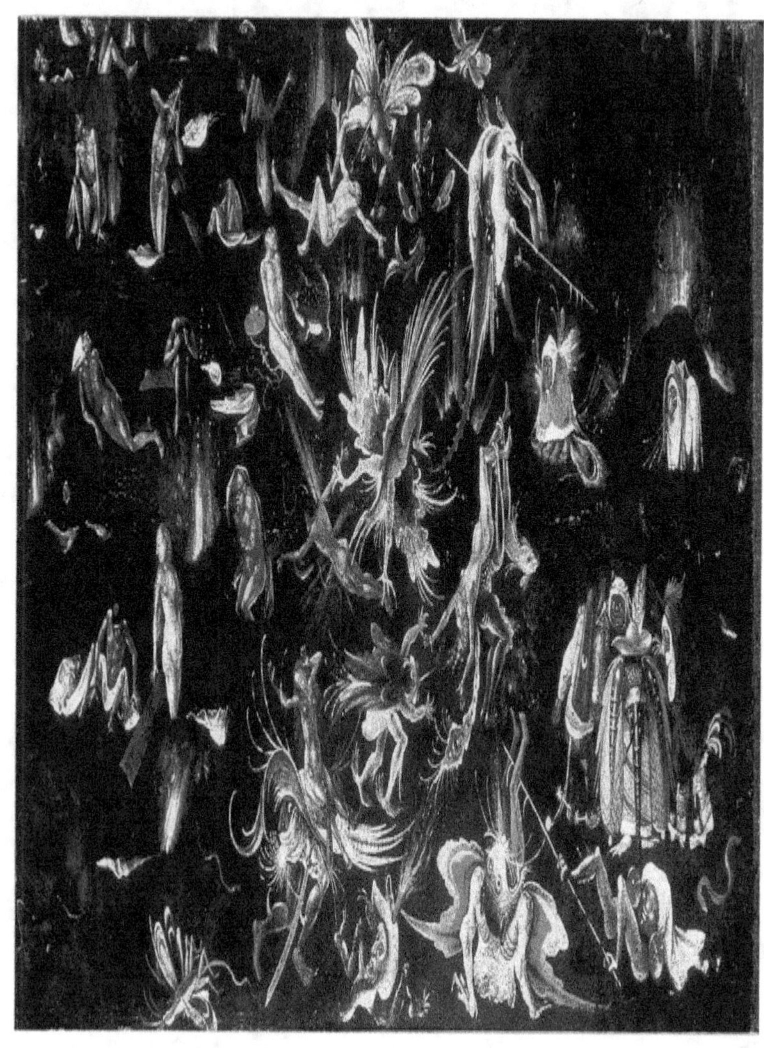

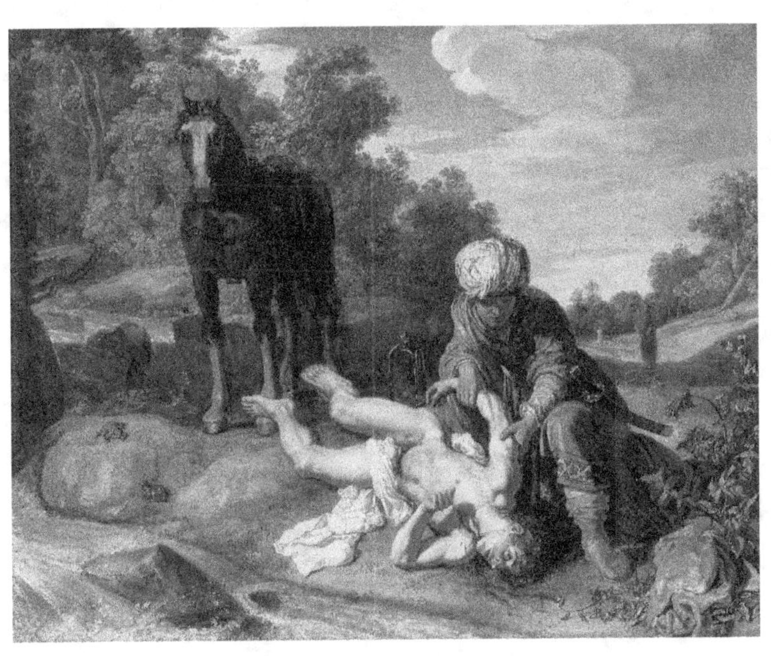

Galatians 5:13-14

...through love be servants to one another. [14] For the whole law is fulfilled in one word, in this: "You shall love your neighbor as yourself."

Breathing Compassion

Bill Briley was known throughout the hospital as the compassionate Respiratory Therapist. While his usual domain was the Intensive Care Unit (ICU), he relished the opportunities to work on other hospital floors. In these settings, he found himself able to engage in meaningful conversations with patients, a luxury often denied to him in the ICU, where most patients were either too sick or connected to machines like BiPAP or ventilators.

In stark contrast to some colleagues who hurried through their rounds to return to their departments or lose themselves in their phones or TVs, Bill approached his work with a dedication to patient care that went beyond the routine. He refused to "stack" treatments, a practice where multiple patients receive treatments simultaneously, preferring instead to give each patient his undivided attention.

When administering inhalation nebulizer treatments, Bill made it a point to stay in the patient's room for the entire duration. As the mist filled the air, he would meticulously review the patient's chart on the computer, analyzing lab results and scrutinizing X-rays of their lungs. If there were signs of improvement, Bill eagerly shared the good news with the patient, presenting them with tangible evidence of their progress. It was a personal touch that even doctors often overlooked in their hurried rounds.

Patients came to appreciate Bill not just for his medical expertise but for his kindness and attention. When the nebulizer treatments concluded, Bill would inquire if there was anything the patient desired – be it ice water, soda, crackers, or peanut butter. By attending to these requests, he not only provided comfort but also lightened the load for the nursing staff, allowing them to focus on their respective responsibilities.

As patients regained their strength and prepared to leave the hospital, Bill took an extra step that set him apart. He would ask if they would like to say a prayer together. In these moments of vulnerability, Bill prayed with the patient and their family, expressing gratitude for the restoration of health. This ritual touched the hearts of many, as it provided solace and a sense of connection during challenging times.

The families of Bill's patients showered him with gratitude, amazed at the depth of care he demonstrated. Bill attributed his approach to the simple philosophy of following God's Golden Rule – treating every patient as he would want to be treated if he were in their position. It was this genuine compassion and unwavering commitment to patient well-being that made Bill Briley a beloved figure in the hospital, leaving a lasting impact on those he cared for.

Breathing Compassion

In the heart of the hospital's hum,

Where illness weaves its tale so glum,

There stood a man of gentle grace,

Bill Briley, with a compassionate embrace.

In ICU's quiet, machines would whir,

Yet Bill yearned for more, a chance to confer.

To other floors, he'd often tread,

Where patients spoke, not machines instead.

No rushing rounds or fleeting glances,

Bill resisted the hurried treatment dances.

No stacking tasks, no hasty retreat,

In each patient's room, he'd take his seat.

Nebulizer mist, a healing fog,

Bill in the room, his eyes agog.

The patient's chart, a story untold,

In data and whispers, a narrative unfold.

Lab results and X-rays, a careful review,
Signs of improvement, a hopeful cue.
Patients' faces lit with joy,
As Bill shared their progress, no time to be coy.

A touch of humanity in the sterile air,
Bill went beyond, showing he cared.
Ice water, soda, crackers, or more,
Comfort he offered, not just a chore.

As patients healed and the time drew near,
To leave the confines, the hospital's sphere.
Bill asked a question, sincere and rare,
"Would you like a prayer, a moment to share?"

He bowed his head, with patients in tow,
A prayer for healing, a comforting glow.
God's Golden Rule, a guiding light,
In Bill's compassion, shining bright.

Families whispered thanks, in awe they'd say,
For Bill's caring touch, in their darkest day.

A Respiratory Therapist, with a heart so vast,

In the tapestry of healing, his kindness cast.

"Breathing Compassion," the title would be,

For Bill's story of care, a poetic decree.

In the corridors where love is spun,

A healer named Bill, whose work is done.

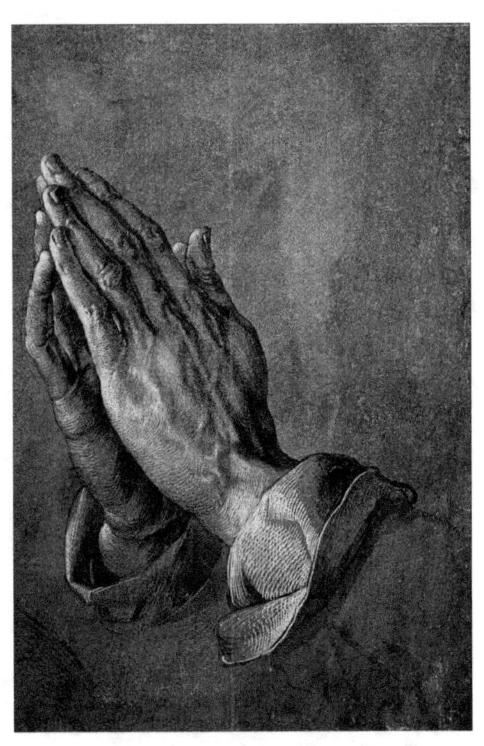

Matthew 7:7-12

Ask, and it will be given you. Seek, and you will find. Knock, and it will be opened for you. 8 For everyone who asks receives. He who seeks finds. To him who knocks it will be opened. 9 Or who is there among you who, if his son asks him for bread, will give him a stone? 10 Or if he asks for a fish, who will give him a serpent? 11 If you then, being sinful in nature, know how to give good gifts to your children, how much more will your Father who is in heaven give good things to those who ask him! **12 Therefore, whatever you desire for men to do to you, you shall also do to them; for this is the law and the prophets.**

Chapter Two

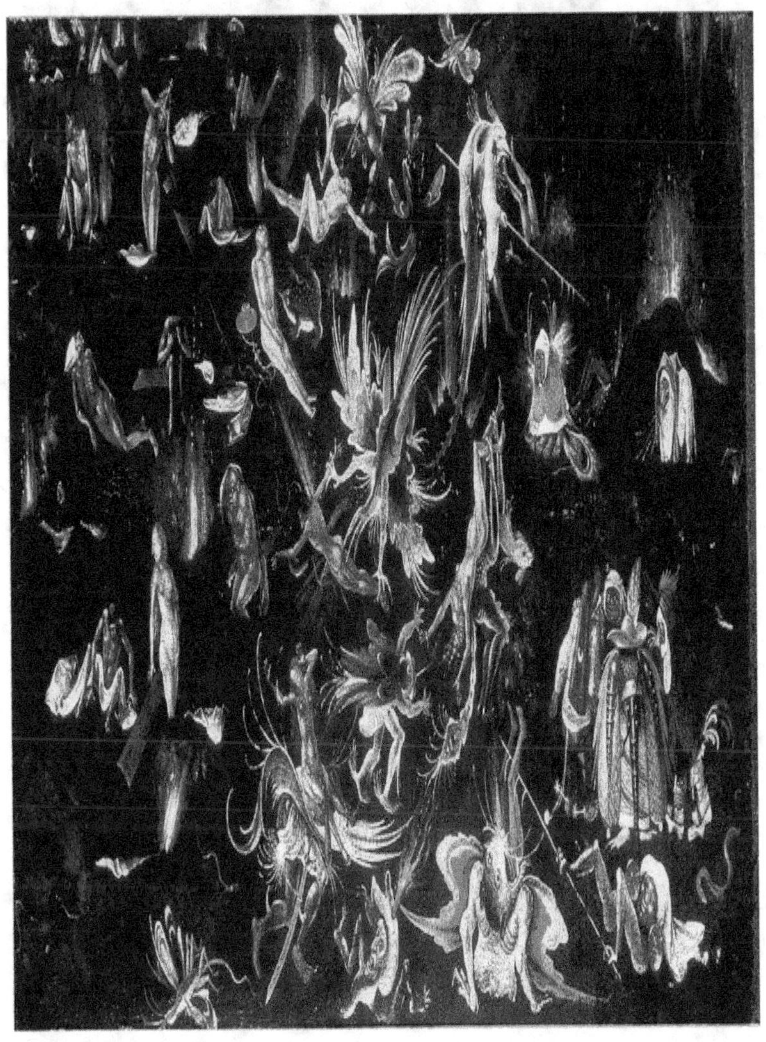

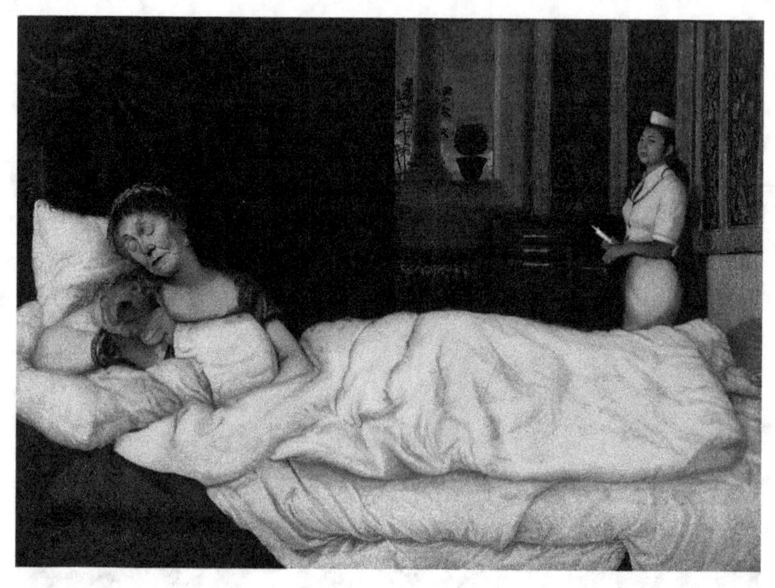

Psalm 41:3

God will sustain them on their sickbed,
and restore them from their bed of illness.

A Breath of Hope

Bill Briley, a seasoned Registered Respiratory Therapist (RRT), found himself on the front lines of the battle against the Covid-19 pandemic, working in a busy hospital ICU in Georgia. He had seen the toll the virus had taken on countless lives, and every day brought new challenges. Bill knew that teamwork and communication were key to providing the best care possible for patients like Mrs. Nana Lopez.

Maria Morales, the bilingual ICU Registered Nurse (RN), was a valuable ally in their fight against the virus. Her fluency in both English and Spanish allowed her to bridge the language gap with many of their Hispanic patients. Today, their patient was Mrs. Nana Lopez, a 64-year-old Covid-19 patient who had been on a BiPAP machine for 24 hours. Despite their best efforts, her condition had worsened, with increasing work of breathing and a continuously dropping SaO2 level, even as the oxygen and BiPAP pressure levels were maxed out.

Bill knew that they needed more accurate data to make informed decisions. He approached Maria and asked her to explain to Nana Lopez, in Spanish, the need for an Arterial Blood Gas (ABG) procedure. The oxygen saturation probe on the patient's finger was a good estimate, but the ABG would provide precise data about her oxygen and carbon dioxide levels. Nana Lopez consented, her eyes reflecting trust in the medical team.

With precision honed through years of experience, Bill carefully drew arterial blood from Nana Lopez's radial artery. The patient remained remarkably composed, not flinching or wincing in response to the small needle. Maria asked if the procedure was painful, and Nana Lopez shook her head, indicating no.

Bill transferred the arterial blood to a portable ABG device, input the required data quickly, and initiated the analysis. The results were grim, indicating severe hypoxemia. Bill knew that immediate action was needed to save Nana Lopez's life.

He paged the ICU doctor assigned to Nana Lopez and informed them of the ABG results. Orders were needed, and they needed to act fast. The doctor's response came swiftly, including the decision to proceed with Endotracheal Tube Intubation and the use of a ventilator.

As Maria explained to Nana Lopez the necessity of intubation, the patient nodded in understanding. She had signed a consent form for this procedure upon her admission to the hospital, fully aware that it might be required to save her life.

With the intubation kit in hand, Bill gathered the tools he needed while also notifying his respiratory therapy teammates through his handsfree headset. Elijah and Jermaine, two skilled colleagues, arrived quickly. Elijah set up the ventilator and oxygenation settings while Jermaine stood by the patient's side.

After Maria administered the sedation medications as ordered, Bill proceeded with the intubation. As he attempted to view the patient's vocal cords, he requested Jermaine to apply cricoid pressure. With their coordinated effort, they achieved success, and the endotracheal tube was successfully inserted. The ventilator was connected, and Bill expressed his gratitude to Elijah, Jermaine, and Maria for their invaluable assistance during this critical procedure.

With Nana Lopez now resting peacefully on the ventilator, her SpO_2 levels registered at a reassuring 98%. After a week on the ventilator, the medical team was able to begin the weaning process. Three long weeks of tireless care and dedication from Bill, his teammates, and Nana Lopez herself led to her recovery. She was finally well enough to return home to her family and loved ones.

Bill, a man of faith, had been praying for Nana Lopez's recovery since the day she arrived in the ICU. As he watched her leave the hospital, he closed his eyes once more, thanking God for answering his prayers as he had done many times in the past. In the midst of a relentless pandemic, this story was a testament to the power of expertise, teamwork, and unwavering hope.

Breath of Hope

In the heart of a battle, in a world undone,
Where a virus rages, and the fight's just begun,
A tale unfolds of courage, of hearts that cope,
In the ICU's embrace, a breath of hope.

Bill, a therapist seasoned, a guardian of air,
With Maria, by his side, a steadfast pair,
Together they stand, to face the storm,
In the COVID ICU, where lives transform.

Nana Lopez, her name a whispered prayer,
Her strength held firm in the suffocating air,
Beneath the mask and the beeping machine,
A story of resilience, yet to be seen.

With SaO2 dropping, her struggle intense,
Bill sought answers, in the midst of suspense,
A small needle, with care, he did employ,
To draw the truth from a silent, willing envoy.

Maria, the bridge, in words so fair,

Explained the need, with a gentle, honest stare,

Consent was granted, and they moved as one,

To unravel the mysteries of what's begun.

Severe hypoxemia, a stark revelation,

Bill paged the doctor, in dire anticipation,

Orders were needed, a battle to be won,

In the name of salvation,

for the patient, Nana Lopez, the chosen one.

Intubation was the path they now must tread,

To save a life hanging by a thread,

With tools and teamwork, they pressed ahead,

A mission to restore the breath that had fled.

With precision and care, in the quiet room,

Bill and his team dispelled the gloom,

The ventilator hummed, with hope it was rife,

And Nana Lopez, in dreams, embraced new life.

Through weeks of toil, and prayers that soared,

The virus's grip, inch by inch, was ignored,

A family's joy, a community's delight,

As Nana Lopez stepped into the healing light.

In the midst of despair, a story took shape,

A symphony of courage, an ode to the great,

In the COVID storm, where shadows elope,

The story of survival, a testament of hope.

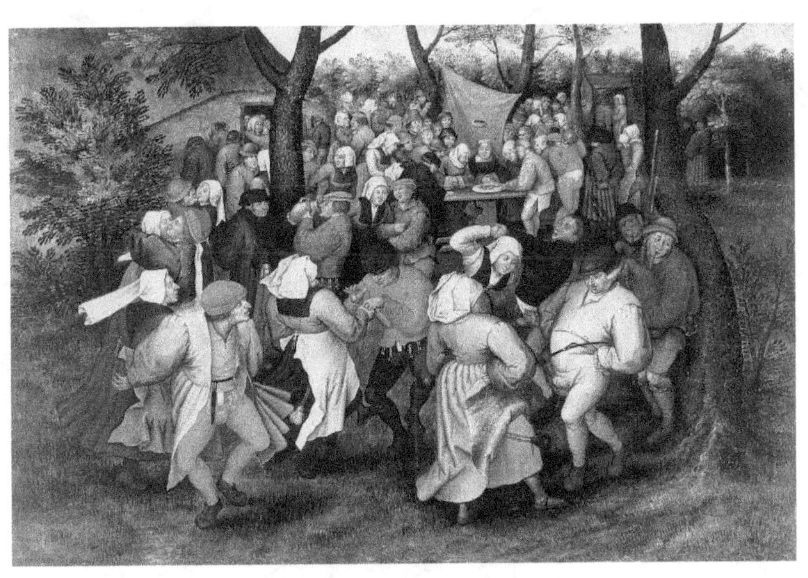

Psalm 150:1-2,6

Praise the Lord!
Praise God in his sanctuary!
Praise him in his heavens for his acts of power!
Praise him for his mighty acts!...
Praise him according to his excellent greatness!
Let everything that has breath praise the Lord!
Praise the Lord!

Chapter Three

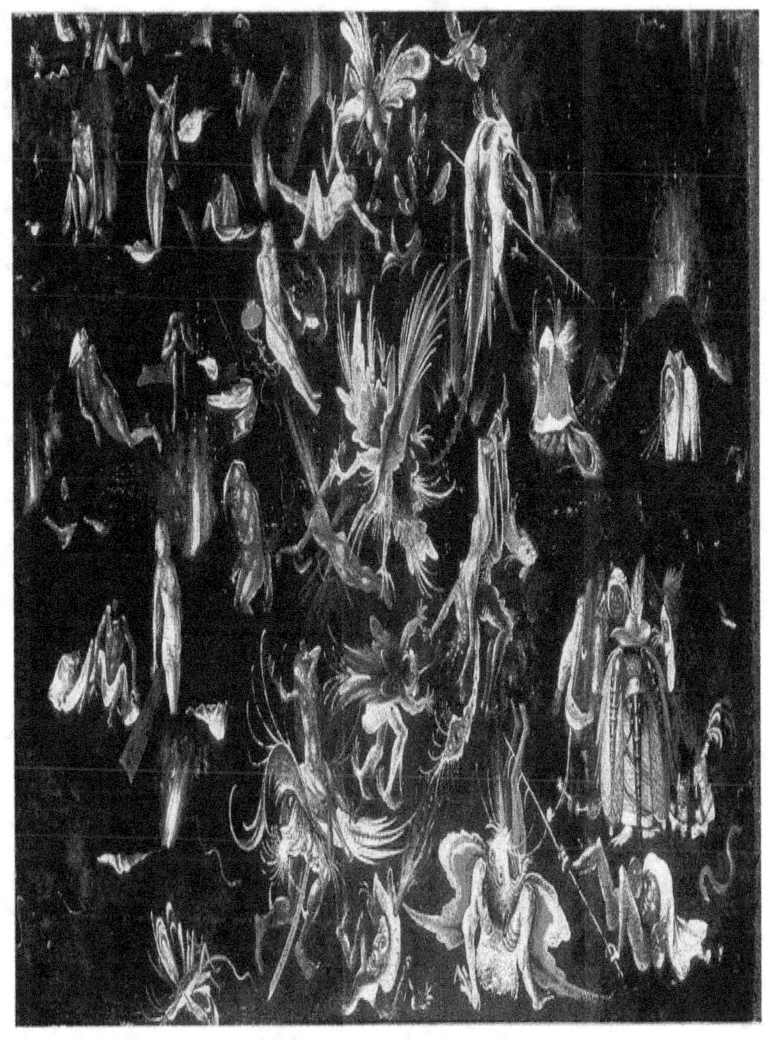

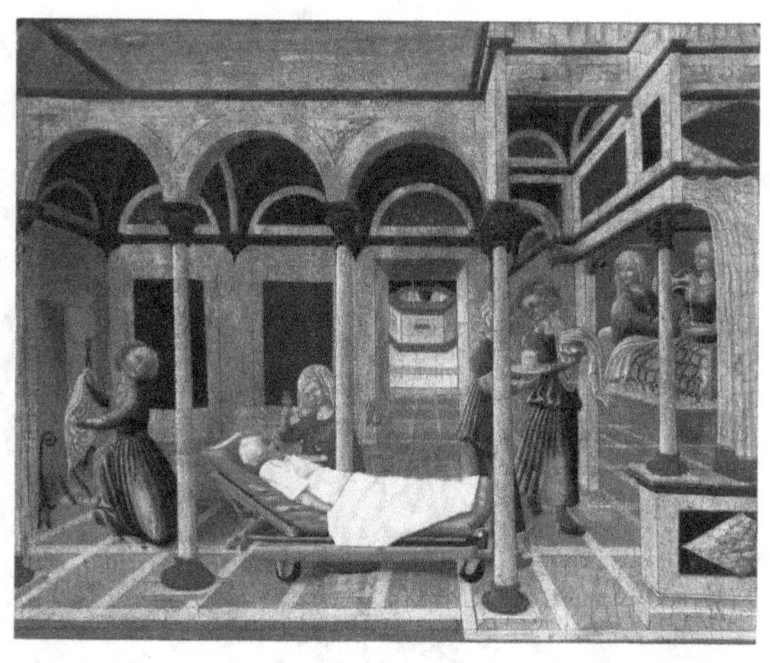

Isaiah 41:10

Don't you be afraid,
for I am with you.
Don't be dismayed,
for I am your God.
I will strengthen you.
Yes, I will help you.
Yes, I will uphold you
with the right hand of
my righteousness.

Icy Water

Respiratory Therapist Bill had just left a chaotic scene on the Med-Surge floor, where a patient's life teetered on the edge, but there was no time for respite. He rushed back to ICU, his footsteps echoing the urgency that coursed through his veins.

The Code Blue button was flashing relentlessly above a Covid-19 patient's room. Bill's heart pounded as he entered, adrenaline surging. He found nurse Lauren struggling to maintain her composure, her gloved hands trembling as she stared at the patient, who was coughing violently, bright red blood gushing into the endotracheal tube connecting the patient to a ventilator.

Time slowed as Bill assessed the situation. With a determined focus, he grabbed a container of ice-cold sterile water, realizing that the bleeding had to stop, and fast. He poured the frigid liquid down the endotracheal tube, which sent a shockwave through the patient's system, causing him to gasp and sputter intermittently.

As the seconds ticked away, Bill continued to flush the tube with cold water, feeling the heat of crisis and the desperate cries of the patient's family outside the door. The blood and mucus, a grotesque mixture, was suctioned out of the tube by Bill. The hemorrhaging stopped as the ice water had effectively forced the capillaries in the lungs to seal.

The room was filled with the tension of life and death, the sound of machines beeping, and the unyielding determination of Bill. Gradually, the coughing subsided, and the bloodletting ceased. Bill's heart raced, but the room was finally filled with a collective sigh of relief.

In the midst of the chaos, Bill had managed to navigate a turbulent sea of blood and despair, ultimately guiding the patient back from the precipice of death. It was a moment of profound significance, where his skills, determination, and the icy, life-saving water had made all the difference.

Icy Water

In the heart of the chaos, Bill stands tall,

His footsteps echo through the hospital hall,

From Med-Surge to ICU, a relentless call,

To save a life, he'll give it his all.

Code Blue flashing, a race against time,

Urgency courses through his veins like a rhyme,

A Covid patient struggles, fighting a climb,

Life and death, on the edge of a dime.

The nurse, trembling, her composure near lost,

Bright red blood, at an alarming cost,

Into the tube, the crimson river crossed,

But Bill's resolve, it will exhaust.

With focus unwavering, he acts in haste,

Sterile water, ice-cold, a life to be chased,

Down the tube, a shockwave, a breath retraced,

In crisis, his determination's embraced.

Seconds tick away, the family outside, they cry,

Machines beeping, life's tethered to the sky,

Blood and mucus, a grotesque lullaby,

Bill's hands steady, never to say goodbye.

Hemorrhaging ceased, the capillaries sealed,

In that icy water, a fate was revealed,

Life's precious thread, in the balance, it wheeled,

In Bill's care, the patient's heart unsealed.

A room once filled with despair and dread,

Now resonates with the breath of life instead,

Machines still hum, but the patient's thread,

Has been rewoven, where hope had nearly fled.

In the midst of chaos, Bill stood tall,

Guided a patient back from the precipice's fall,

With skills and ice water, he answered the call,

In this tale of crisis, where heroes enthrall.

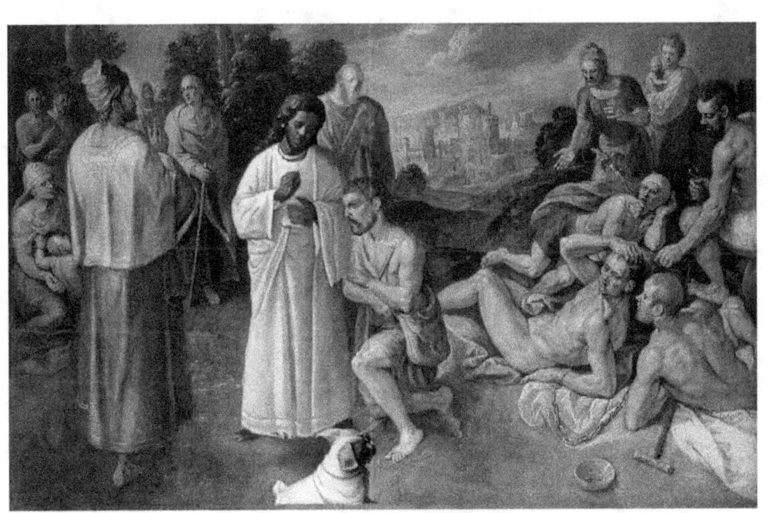

Jeremiah 30:17

*"For I will restore health to you,
and I will heal you of your wounds,"
says the LORD.*

Chapter Four

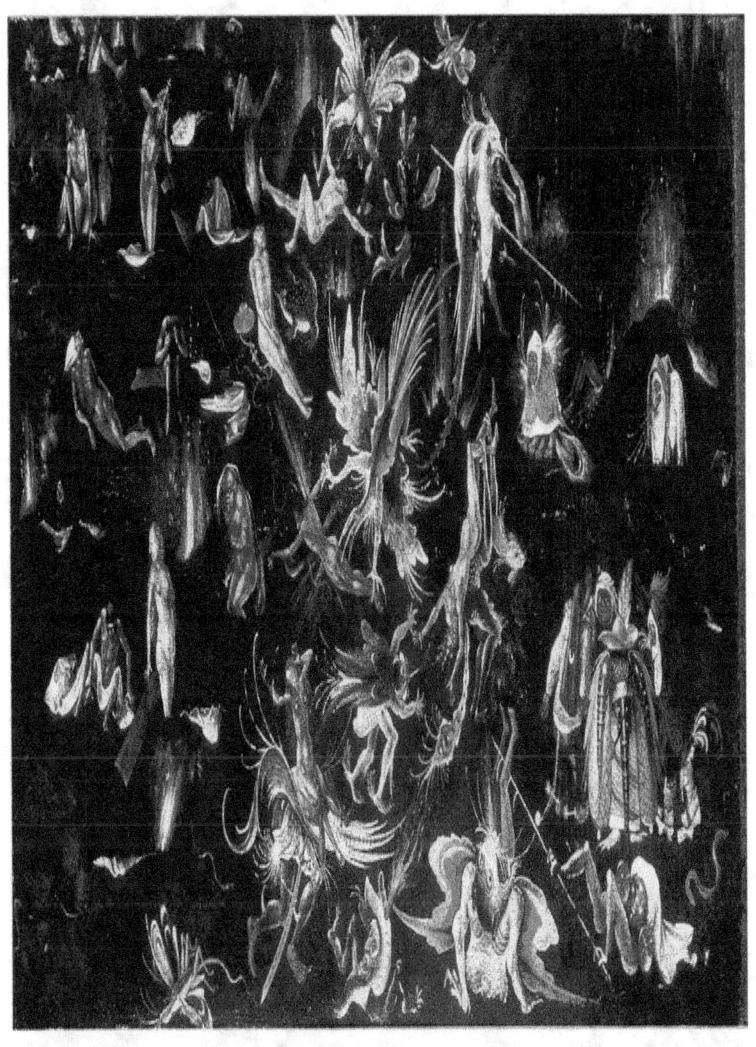

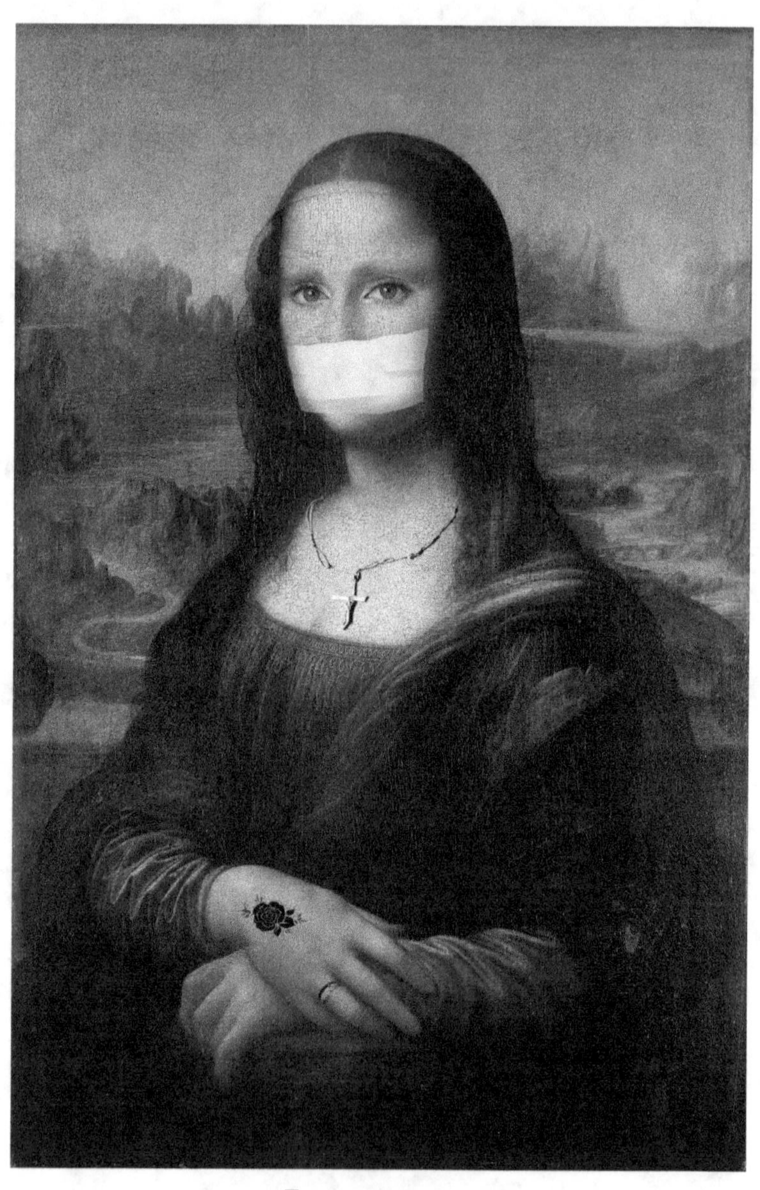

James 4:10

*Humble yourselves in the sight of the Lord,
and he will lift you up.*

A Bond Born in Crisis

In the heart of the storm, amidst the pandemic's strife, the world witnessed a bond that would forever change the lives of two remarkable individuals, Bill and Maria. They were thrust into the front lines of the battle against a relentless enemy, working side by side in the intensive care unit of a bustling hospital.

As the virus surged, so did the demand for dedicated healthcare professionals. Bill, a seasoned Respiratory Therapist with a heart full of compassion, had always been the quiet hero, working tirelessly to ensure that his patients could breathe and fight for another day. Maria, a young and spirited nurse, had a smile that could light up even the darkest of days, and her unwavering dedication to her patients was a source of inspiration for everyone around her.

The hospital's ICU had become a battlefield, where they fought not against another army but against an invisible foe that had brought the world to its knees. Patients flooded in, their breaths labored, their fear palpable. It was amidst this chaos that Bill and Maria found themselves, their lives entwined by their shared mission to save others.

They shared long shifts, donned in layers of PPE that concealed their faces but not their unwavering commitment. As the virus raged on, they witnessed moments of heartbreak and hope in equal measure. They held the hands of the dying, provided solace to the grieving, and celebrated every small victory with smiles hidden beneath their masks.

In those trying times, a bond was forged that transcended the confines of the hospital walls. They found strength in each other's presence; their teamwork unwavering. Bill's expertise with the ventilators was complemented by Maria's tender care and comforting words to patients. Their courage and compassion became a beacon of hope in the darkest of lands, reminding everyone that even in the face of a pandemic, humanity's light could shine through.

Their journey was far from easy, and the toll it took on them was immeasurable. They were heroes, not just because of the lives they saved but because of the sacrifices they made. They were bound by a shared purpose, a shared resilience that no pandemic could break.

As the storm began to subside, and antiviral medications offered a glimmer of hope, Bill and Maria looked back on their shared odyssey. They had faced the storm head-on, their bond growing stronger with each passing day. Their story became a testament to the unwavering spirit of healthcare workers, who selflessly stood at the forefront of the crisis, ensuring that the flame of humanity burned bright even in the darkest hours.

A Bond Born in Crisis

In the heart of the storm, 'midst

the pandemic's strife,

Two heroes emerged, Bill and

Maria, in the fight for life.

In the hospital's ICU, they bore

the burden, hand in hand,

Their courage and compassion,

a light in the darkest land.

Bill, with stethoscope and

Steady hands so wise,

Maria, with her nurturing soul

And empathetic eyes,

Together they stood,

Unwavering against the tide,

Their hearts bound by a

Purpose, compassion as their

Guide.

Through long and trying shifts,

And the tears they couldn't hide,

They found a kindred spirit,

Right there by their side.

In the beeping of monitors, they

Heard a common song,

In the faces behind masks, they

Found where they belong.

They shared stories of patients,

Each triumph, and each fail,

Through the pain and sorrow,

They gave it their all.

As the world seemed to

Crumble, and fear was all

Around,

Bill and Maria's friendship was on

Solid ground.

They faced exhaustion and

Despair, but they never let go,

Their strength as a team would

Forever glow.

Through the worst of those

Years, 'neath the pandemic's

Strain,

A lifelong bond was forged, and

It would remain.

In the end, when the chaos

Began to recede,

Bill and Maria, united in their

Noble deed,

From those ICU days to a future

Yet untold,

Their friendship a testament, a

Love that will never grow old.

Through the darkness of the

Pandemic, their spirits did

Mend,

Bill and Maria, two heroes,

Forever friends.

In the hospital's ICU, where their

Spirits did ascend,

They found the light in each
Other, a *friendship* without end.

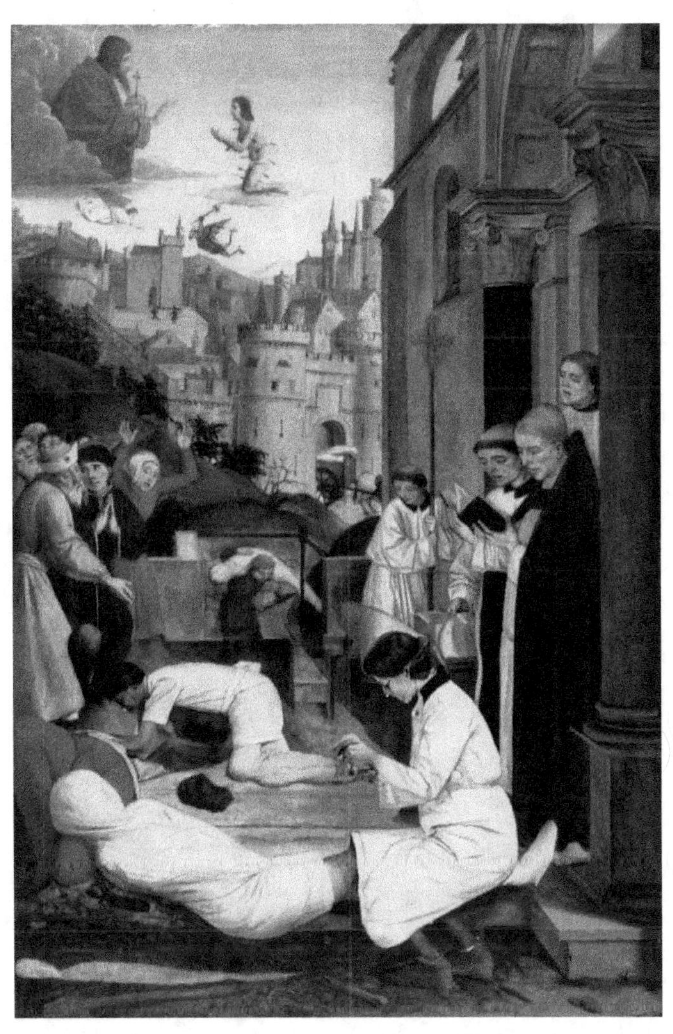

Ecclesiastes 4:9-10

Two are better than one, because they have a good reward for their labor. ¹⁰ For if they fall, the one will lift up his friend; but woe to him who is alone when he falls, and doesn't have another to lift him up.

Chapter Five

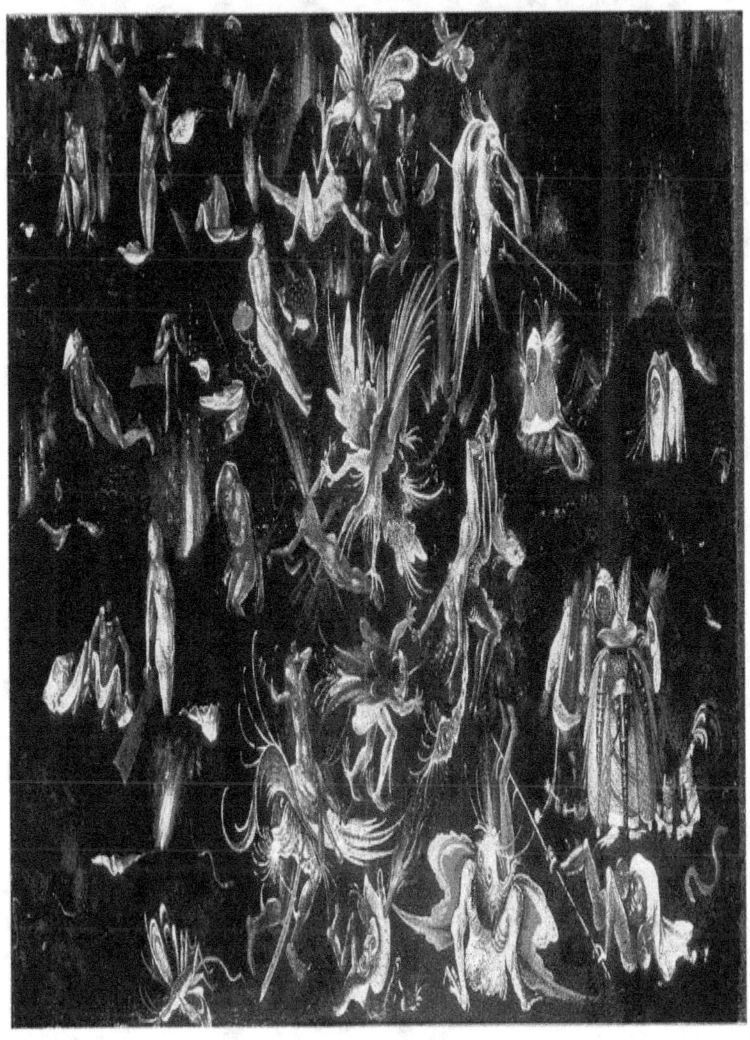

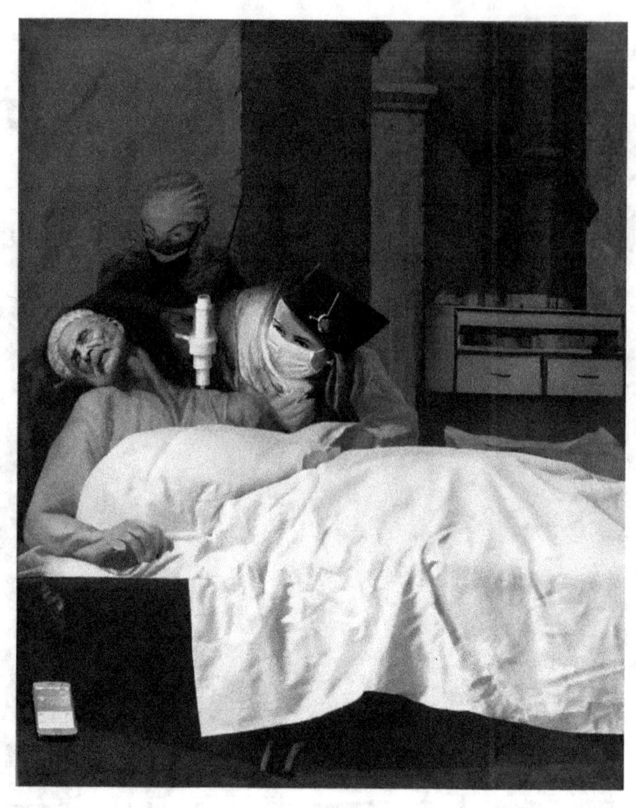

Psalm 34:17-19

The righteous cry, and the LORD hears, and delivers them out of all their troubles. 18 The LORD is near to those who have a broken heart, and saves those who have a crushed spirit. 19 Many are the afflictions of the righteous, but the LORD delivers him out of them all.

COVID's Tricks Can Cloud a Mind

In the heart of the bustling hospital, in a sterile room of the intensive care unit, Bill, the dedicated Respiratory Therapist, and Maria, the compassionate nurse, were accustomed to the daily struggles of treating COVID-19 patients. Their spirits may have been worn thin, but their determination remained unshaken.

One gloomy morning, Bill pushed the door to Room 312 ajar and walked in, carrying a nebulizer in hand. There lay an elderly man, Jasper Bedford, his face etched with lines of worry, his eyes red and brimming with tears. The soft hum of the machines was interrupted only by Jasper Bedford's quiet sobs.

With empathy in his voice, Bill asked, "Jasper, what's troubling you today? How can I help?"

The elderly man, struggling to catch his breath, managed to whisper, "My wife...she's...she's leaving me."

Bill set the nebulizer aside and pulled a chair closer to the bed. He gently inquired, "Why do you think that, Jasper? I'm sure there's a misunderstanding."

With a heavy sigh, Jasper began to recount the story. "We've been married for fifty years, you see. But she's on the Med-Surge floor, and I talked to her on the phone today. She said she wanted a divorce. I can't bear to lose her after all these years."

Maria, who had been silently observing from the corner of the room, joined the conversation. "Jasper, COVID can sometimes affect a person's brain, making them disoriented. Your wife might not even realize what she's saying right now. It's the virus playing tricks on her mind."

Tears welled up in Jasper's eyes, and he nodded, taking some comfort in the explanation. "You think so?"

Bill nodded reassuringly. "Absolutely. Once she recovers, she'll be back to her old self, and she'll remember how much you mean to her. In the meantime, let's keep you strong, so you can be there for her."

For the next week, Bill and Maria made it a point to visit Jasper daily. They administered his Albuterol treatments and offered words of encouragement. Despite his fragile state, they saw a spark of hope in his eyes with every visit.

Then, one sunny morning, Bill walked into Room 312, expecting to find the same worried and downtrodden Jasper. Instead, there was a sight he had never anticipated. Jasper was grinning from ear to ear, his eyes twinkling with joy.

"Jasper, you look fantastic today," Bill exclaimed.

The elderly man's laughter was like music. "You won't believe it, Bill. My wife called me this morning. She said she loves me and has no memory of wanting a divorce when she was sick. She's getting better!"

Tears of joy welled up in Jasper's eyes, this time not out of sadness but pure happiness. Maria, who had joined Bill, beamed with joy, too.

Bill patted Jasper's shoulder. "See, I told you, Jasper, love is stronger than any illness. It's a beautiful thing to witness."

Maria added, "We'll keep working hard to make sure you both recover fully, and soon, you'll be holding each other's hands once more."

Jasper Bedford nodded and clutched the phone in his hand. His smile was brighter than ever as he looked out the window at the world beyond. He had weathered the storm with the support of two caring individuals, and his love story was far from over.

COVID's Tricks Can Cloud a Mind

Amid the bustling hospital's relentless pace,

In the ICU, where courage they embrace,

Bill and Maria, their steps in the race,

Daily struggles etched on their steadfast face.

Their spirits, weathered, but resolve intact,

Facing COVID's storm, no spirit lacked,

A gloomy morn, a patient's heart was cracked,

In Room 312, where hope seemed sacked.

An elderly man, Jasper Bedford's name,

Worries etched upon his face, his frame,

Bill entered gently, in the illness's flame,

To heal not just the body, but the soul's reclaim.

"Jasper, tell me what ails your heart,

In this sterile room, a world apart,

Your love's at stake, torn apart,

How can I assist, where can I start?"

Jasper Bedford, whispered through his tears,

Of fifty years, of love's lingering fears,

"She's leaving," his voice trembled with years,

The words, a torrent of pain, his heart's frontiers.

Bill pulled a chair and shared a caring word,

Embracing the man whose love seemed absurd,

Maria stood in silence, her presence heard,

In the corner, compassion was conferred.

"COVID's tricks can cloud a mind,

A loving heart, sometimes it blinds,

Your wife's disoriented, please be kind,

In her heart, your love she'll find."

Comforted by their words, Jasper sighed,

Hope, like a glimmer, he could not hide,

Bill, Maria, by his side,

In that moment, a bond, a healing tide.

For days they cared, in his room they'd stand,

The nebulizer's hiss, a healing hand,

In the fragility, where strength was planned,

A spark of hope, in Jasper Bedford, fanned.

Then, one morning, a radiant delight,

In Room 312, a wondrous sight,

Jasper Bedford's eyes, so wide and bright,

He was no longer lost in the night.

"Bill, she loves me, can it be true?"

His laughter, like music, as morning dew,

In their hearts, the joy steadily grew,

Bill and Maria, the dream's debut.

Love, the beacon through the tempest's rain,

In a hospital room, healing the pain,

Bill and Maria, a steadfast chain,

In the heart of the hospital's grace, love's terrain.

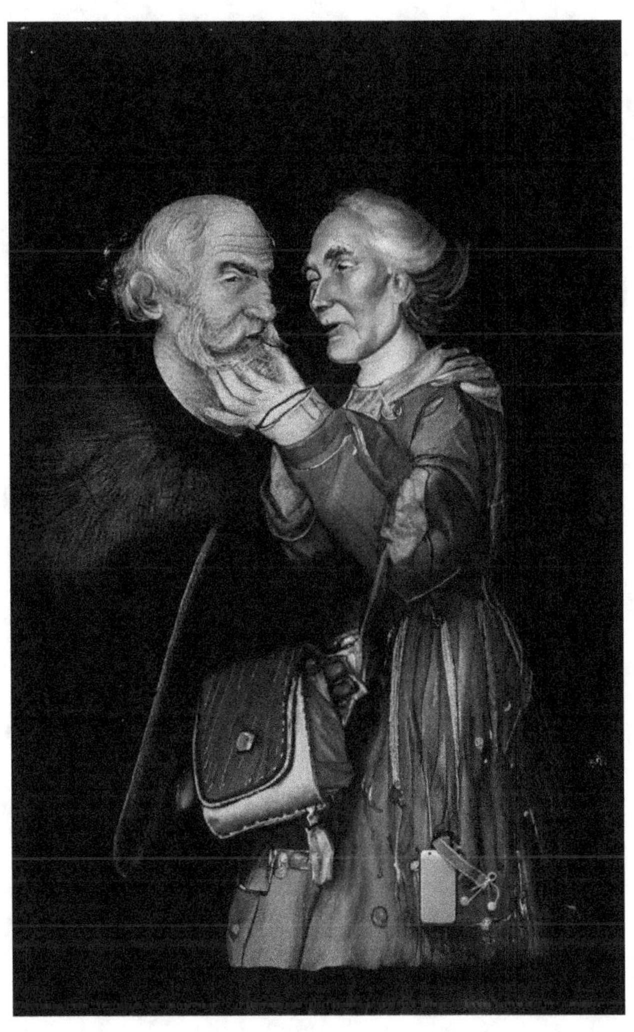

Ephesians 4:1-2

I therefore, a servant of the Lord, beg you to walk worthily of the calling with which you were called, 2 with all lowliness and humility, with patience, bearing with one another in love.

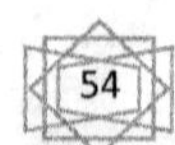

Chapter Six

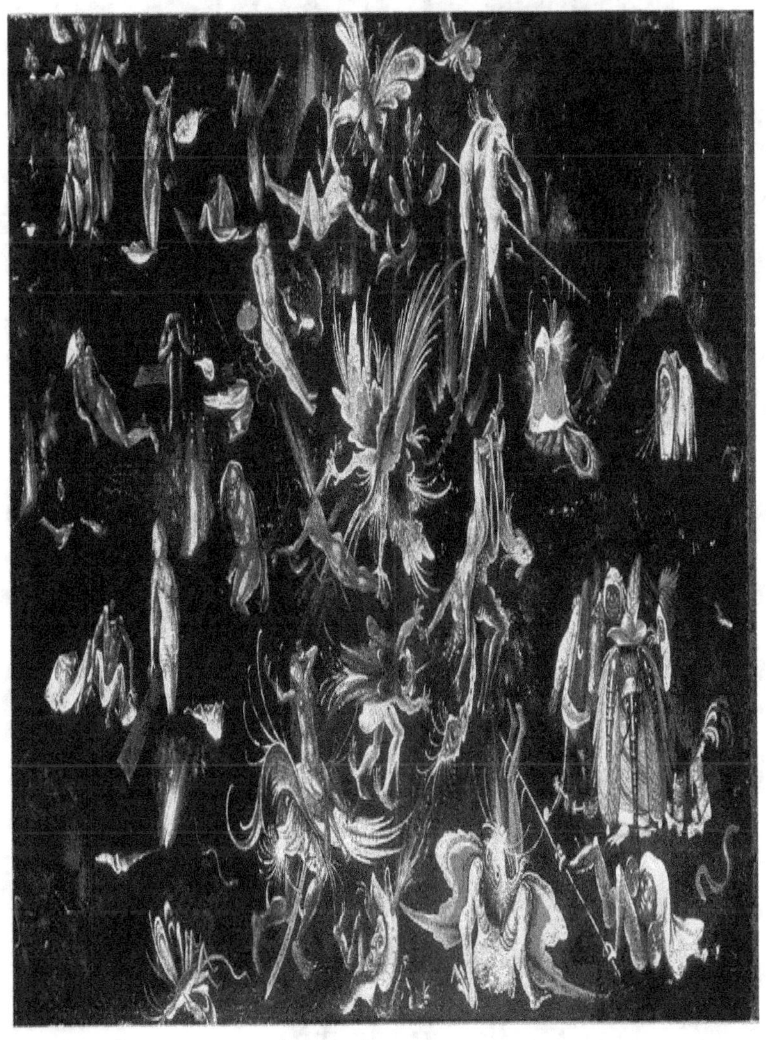

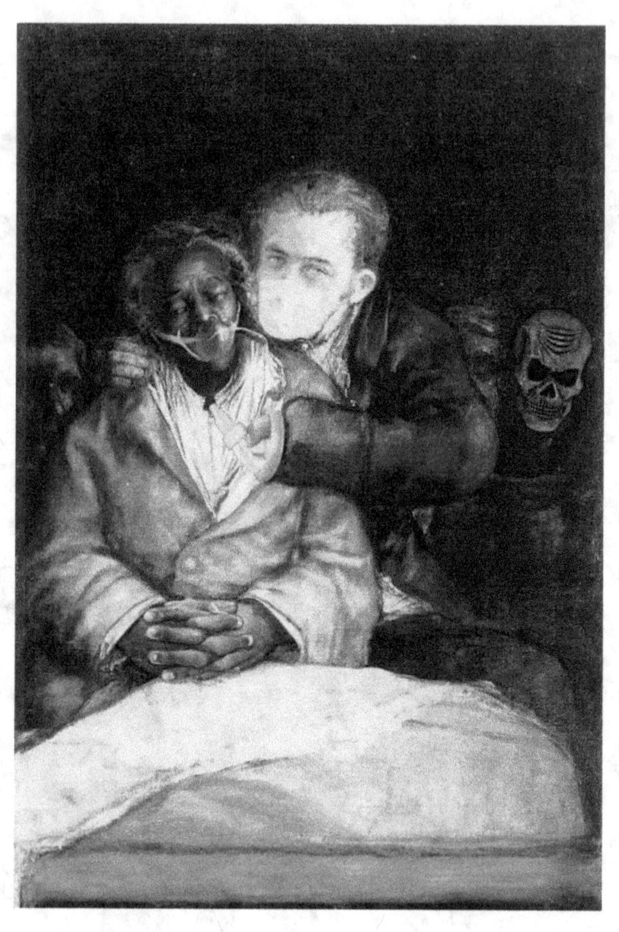

Isaiah 38:14

...My eyes weaken looking upward.
Lord, I am crushed.
Be my security.

Breathing Life

In the dimly lit intensive care unit of the bustling city hospital, Bill, the dedicated Respiratory Therapist, embarked on another grueling 12-hour shift. The sun had yet to rise as he prepared to perform a weaning trial on a patient who had become a symbol of resilience during the trying times of the Covid-19 pandemic. Deshaun Douglas, a 57-year-old husband and father of five children, had been clinging to life on a ventilator for the past three weeks.

Deshaun's journey had been fraught with uncertainty, his condition near death when he first arrived at the ICU. But thanks to the unwavering dedication of Bill and his team, along with a myriad of trial medications, the relentless Covid-19 virus within Deshaun had been gradually eradicated. The previous day, the virus was no longer detected in his body, bringing a glimmer of hope to his family who had been living through this harrowing ordeal.

Deshaun's daily routine consisted of being turned from supine to prone and back every 12 hours to optimize oxygenation. In the first week, Bill and his colleagues had even performed a Bronchoscopy to remove thick secretions from deep within Deshaun's bronchi. His path to recovery had been filled with ups and downs, but today was a special day, one filled with anticipation and anxiety, for it was the day Bill would run the final weaning trial on the ventilator to determine if Deshaun was strong enough to breathe on his own.

Deshaun had already been on a sedation vacation, a process where the medications that had kept him sedated during the night were turned off, allowing him to gradually wake up. He could now hear and respond to Bill, forming a connection beyond the cold, life-sustaining machinery surrounding him.

With a gentle smile and words of encouragement, Bill began the weaning trial, gradually reducing the pressure support provided by the ventilator. Every moment was filled with tension, as Bill carefully monitored Deshaun's vital signs. The room was silent, except for the soft hissing of the ventilator, as Deshaun's chest rose and fell with every breath.

Miraculously, Deshaun Douglas was able to breathe without the assistance of the ventilator during the weaning trial. His body was now strong enough to take the next step on his journey to recovery. With a sense of triumph and relief, Bill prepared to execute the extubation procedure. He had already received the necessary orders, and with skilled hands, he gently removed the endotracheal tube from Deshaun's trachea, finally silencing the machine that had been his lifeline for so long.

As the ventilator stood on standby, Bill turned to Deshaun with tears of joy in his eyes. He patted Deshaun's shoulder and spoke words of hope and happiness. "You've conquered Covid, Deshaun," he said, "and you'll be going home to your wife and children soon."

Deshaun's eyes twinkled with gratitude and joy, a silent testimony to the resilience of the human spirit.

Bill, overwhelmed with emotion, reached for his phone and dialed the number he knew by heart – Deshaun's family. As he delivered the wonderful news, Deshaun's wife's voice trembled with relief and gratitude. She thanked Bill for being a guardian angel who had played a crucial role in saving her beloved husband and the father of their children.

Bill felt his heart swell with love and compassion for this family. After the call, he bowed his head and said a silent prayer to the heavens, thanking God for the miracle of healing he had been part of. In a world marred by the pandemic, Bill's dedication and the resilience of Deshaun Douglas became a beacon of hope, reminding everyone that, even in the darkest of times, there is room for miracles, compassion, and the unwavering dedication of individuals like Bill.

Breathing Life

In the ICU's silent realm so stark,

Where battle cries wage in the dark,

Bill the healer with unwavering heart,

Championed life, played his part.

Before the sun's first golden ray,

Bill began his grueling day,

With Deshaun's fight held in his sway,

In a world where shadows lay.

Deshaun, a father with dreams untold,

Once lay near death, his spirit bold,

Covid's grip on his life took hold,

As Bill's devotion steadily unfold.

Weeks turned days, hope a fragile spark,

The virus fading from Deshaun's mark,

From supine to prone, they danced the dark,

Bill and team, a healing ark.

Bronchoscopy, their hands did guide,

To remove the secrets deep inside,

A family's love as their guide,

In the turbulent, life's wild ride.

The trial arrived, a moment of grace,

Deshaun met Bill, a gentle face,

Whispered words in that sacred space,

As the ventilator slowed its pace.

Bill's skilled hand, a master's touch,

Reduced the pressure, oh so much,

Deshaun's breath, a trembling clutch,

In the silence, they did clutch.

The ventilator stood aside,

As Bill removed what did confide,

The tube that bound, the lifeline tied,

Deshaun's spirit, no longer denied.

In that room of tears and gleam,

Deshaun's eyes with a hopeful beam,

Bill, the healer, part of the dream,

A whispered prayer, in love, they scheme.

"Breathing Life," the story's name,

In the ICU's relentless game,

A testament to Bill's gentle flame,

Where hope and love forever claim.

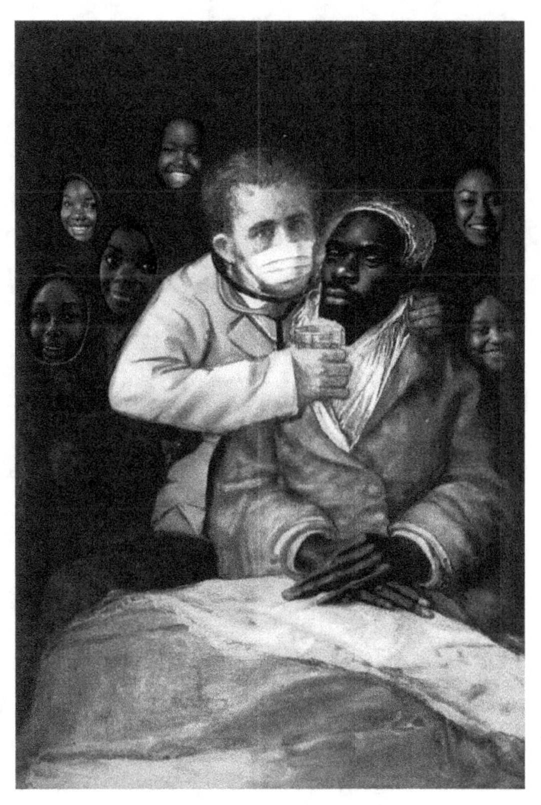

Isaiah 38:20

The LORD will save me!

Philippians 4:4

Rejoice in the Lord always!
Again, I will say, "Rejoice!"

Chapter Seven

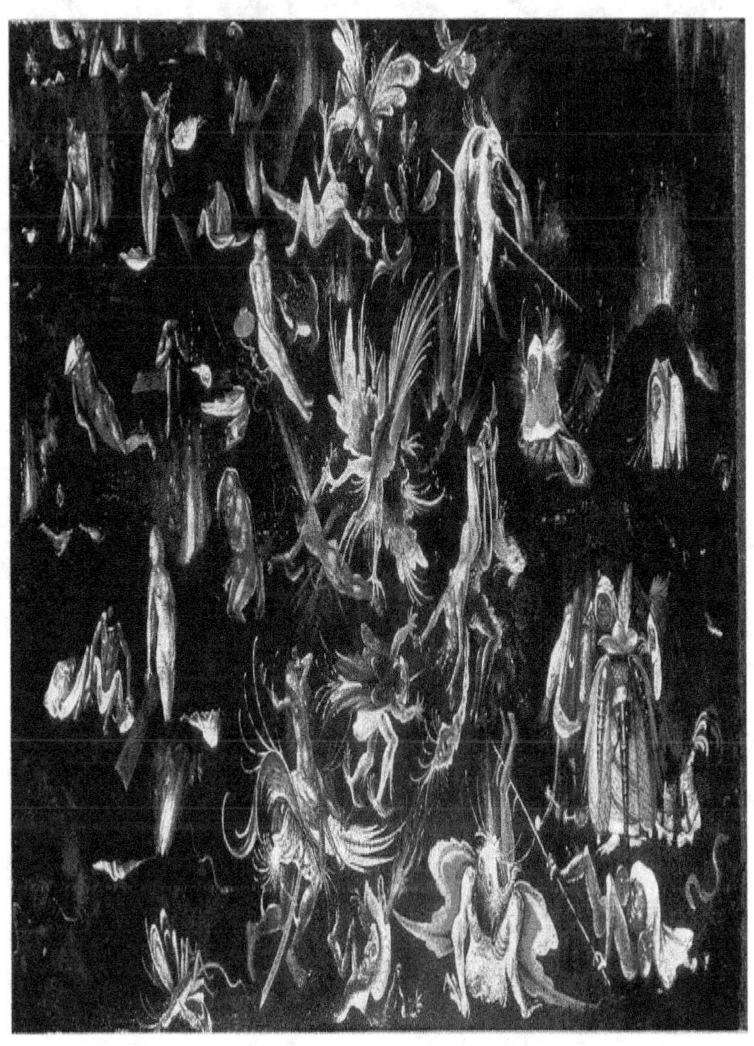

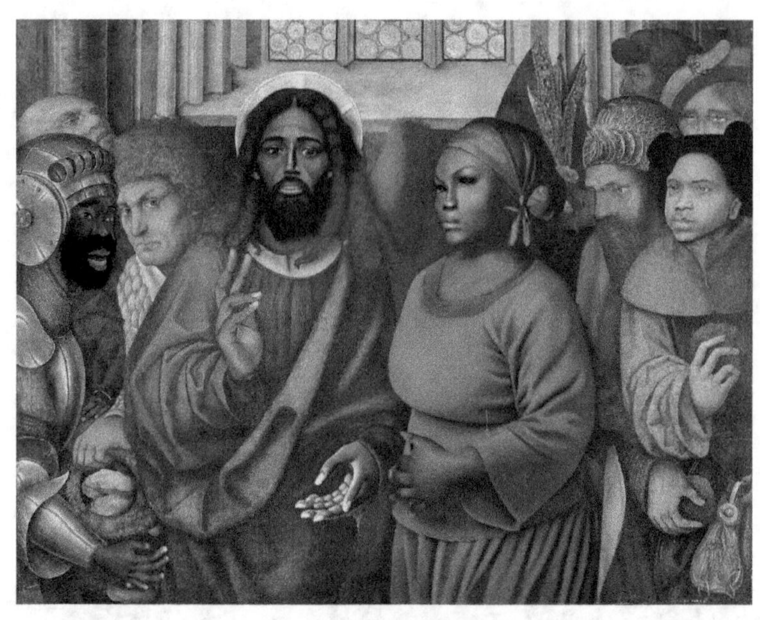

Proverbs 27:17

Iron sharpens iron;
so a man sharpens
his friend's countenance.

Remembering Lashunda

Amid the thriving metropolis of Atlanta, the COVID-19 pandemic had unleashed its wrath on the local hospital, where Bill worked as a dedicated Respiratory Therapist. Each day, he donned his personal protective equipment (PPE) and stepped into the intensive care unit, facing the relentless wave of patients battling the virus. Among the hospital staff was a young, compassionate woman named Lashunda, who worked as a certified nursing assistant (CNA) on one of the quarantined floors.

Lashunda was a symbol of resilience in the face of adversity. She had diabetes and was extremely overweight, factors that made her particularly vulnerable to the virus. Yet, she continued to work diligently, caring for patients, even as the virus raged on.

As the first wave of COVID-19 began to wane, there was a sense of relief, perhaps even complacency, that swept through the hospital. Some staff members believed that the worst was over, and the risk of contracting the virus had diminished. However, the Infection Control department continually reminded the medical teams, including the Respiratory Therapists, nurses, and CNAs, that the battle was far from won. They emphasized the importance of unwavering vigilancc, always donning PPE when entering a patient's room.

But tragedy is a relentless force of its own. Despite the ongoing safety measures, Lashunda contracted COVID-19. The virus wreaked havoc on her body, and soon, she required ventilator support in the very ICU where she had once provided care. The sight of Lashunda, lying helplessly in the same place she had dedicated herself to, sent shockwaves through the hospital staff, including Bill. They fought tirelessly, but the virus had claimed a fellow warrior.

In the dimly lit ICU, the hospital staff witnessed a heart-wrenching scene as Lashunda's parents visited her, their faces etched with pain and disbelief. They held her hand, whispered words of love and comfort, but their daughter could no longer respond. The room seemed to hold the weight of an entire community's grief, and the loss of a dedicated young woman, who had served with unwavering compassion, left an indelible mark on the hearts of her colleagues.

Lashunda's tragic passing served as a stark reminder that the battle against COVID-19 was far from over, and that the virus could strike even the most dedicated and diligent healthcare workers. As Bill continued to care for patients in the ICU, he carried the memory of Lashunda's sacrifice, a testament to the relentless and often unpredictable nature of the pandemic. Her story was a painful reminder that while the world yearned for a return to normalcy, the fight against COVID-19 required unwavering vigilance, resilience, and unity.

Remembering Lashunda

Amid Atlanta's thriving heart, a tale unfolds,

A pandemic's grip, where countless stories told,

Bill, a beacon, his PPE like gold,

In the ICU, a battlefield bold.

In this metropolis, where hopes were high,

Where heroes donned their armor, touched the sky,

Lashunda's presence, a resolute ally,

In the face of darkness, she dared to defy.

A CNA with strength, her heart so vast,

Vulnerable to the virus's ruthless blast,

Yet, she stood firm, holding steadfast,

In her care, compassion, unsurpassed.

As the pandemic's first wave began to fade,

Relief surged forth, like a serenade,

But in the shadows, danger had not swayed,

The virus, a foe, still unafraid.

In the hospital's corridors, they fought,

Against complacency, the lessons they sought,

Infection Control's voice, a warning thought,

To don PPE, was the rule they'd be taught.

But tragedy, relentless, had its say,

Lashunda caught the virus one fateful day,

In the ICU, she lay, where once she'd stay,

A CNA in need, life's colors turned gray.

Her body ravaged, the virus took its course,

Ventilator's hum, a lifeline, no remorse,

The battle within, a turbulent force,

In Lashunda's honor, they'd stay the course.

In dim-lit ICU, a scene so stark,

Colleagues bore the weight of grief's dark mark,

Her parents' visit, a pain so stark,

In their whispers, love's eternal spark.

Lashunda's sacrifice, a painful cost,

Her dedication, humanity's embossed,

In the hearts of her colleagues, never to be lost,

A memory of a hero, despite the tempest's frost.

A stark reminder, the battle's far from done,

The virus relentless, no battles won,

In unity, resilience, they'd see the sun,

Lashunda's legacy, to everyone, a solemn one.

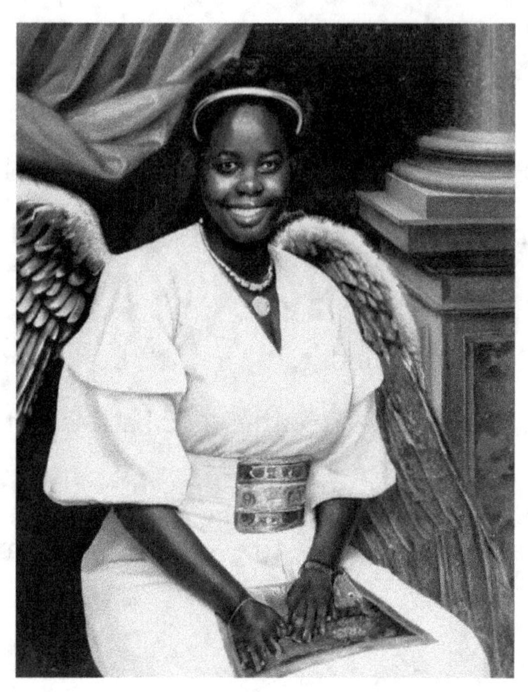

Matthew 5:10

*Blessed are those who are martyrs
For the sake of righteousness,
For theirs is
The kingdom of heaven.*

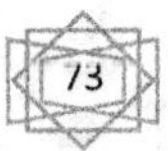

Chapter Eight

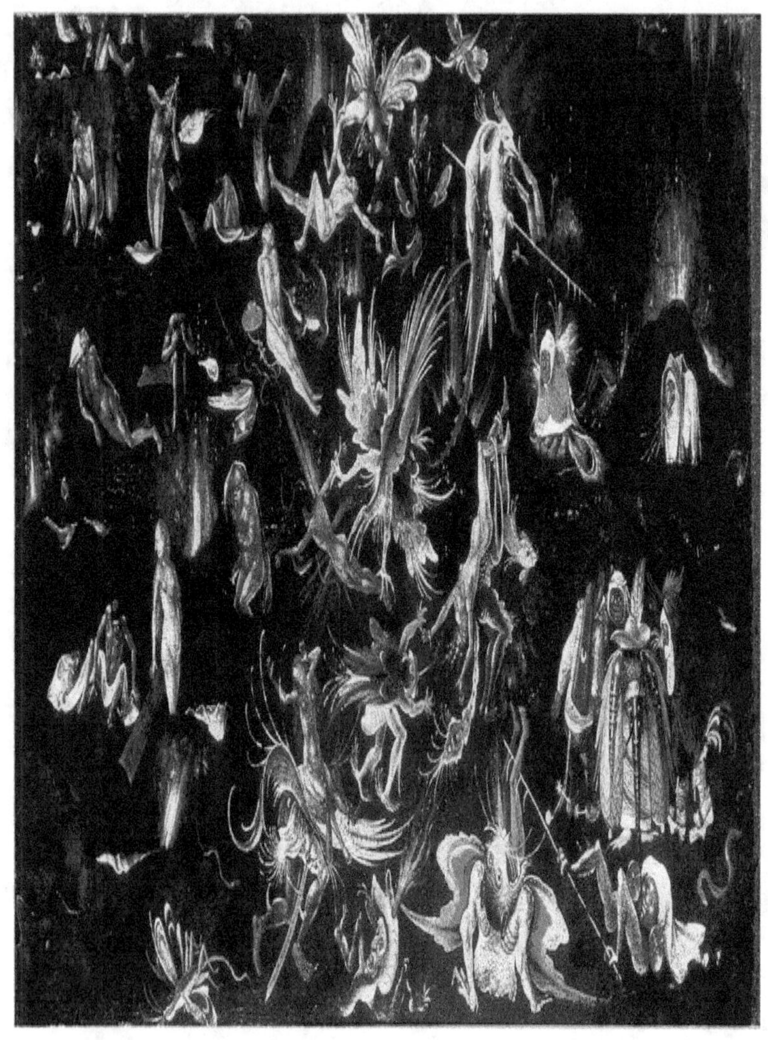

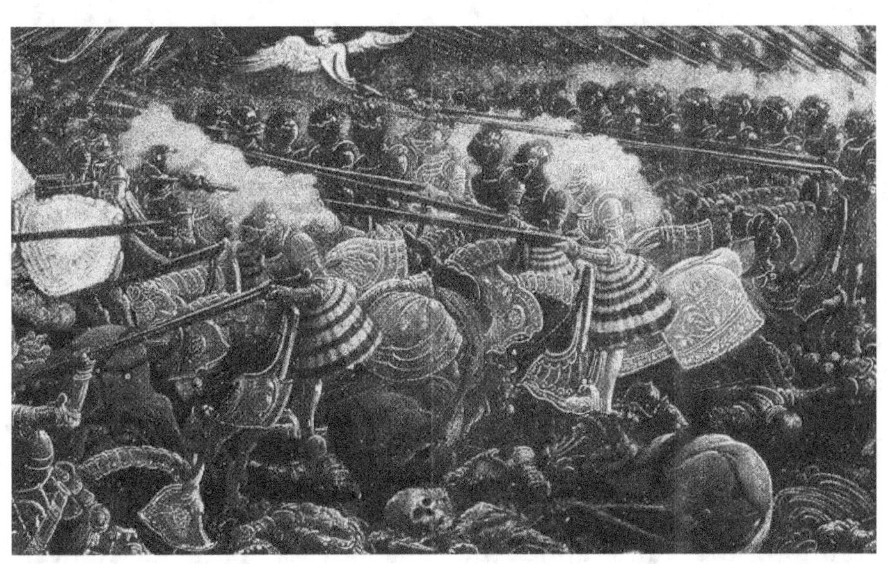

Mark 3:35

*Whoever does God's will
is my brother...*

Proverbs 17:17

*A friend loves at all times;
and a brother is born for adversity.*

Brothers of the
Pandemic Frontline

In the heart of the hellscape that had become the hospital's COVID-19 battleground, a band of brothers emerged, bound not by blood but by their shared purpose and unyielding determination. Among them was Bill, a dedicated Respiratory Therapist, whose unwavering resolve was matched only by his desire to save lives.

Jermaine, the elder statesman of the group, commanded respect like no other. His wealth of knowledge and expertise was renowned, particularly in the emergency arena. He was a master of intubation, the calm amid the chaos when patients went into respiratory distress. In the darkest hours of the night, his presence brought reassurance, as he navigated the complexities of critical cases with the grace of a seasoned captain.

Elijah, the young college professor turned traveling Respiratory Therapist, was a shining star in their midst. Hailing from South Carolina, he embodied the spirit of resilience. His schedule was relentless, a grueling 12-hour shift, five to six days a week, with only a few precious moments of rest in between. Yet, somehow, Elijah found the strength and conviction to make it to the gym several times each week. His determination was infectious, and it was a force that would change lives.

Bill, who had battled his own personal struggles, admired Elijah's unwavering commitment to both his patients and his health. Their camaraderie grew as the two spent countless hours side by side, managing ventilators and ensuring the critically ill received the care they needed. The conversations between shifts revolved not only around cases and patient progress but also around diet, exercise, and well-being.

Over the course of two years, as they shared the front lines of this relentless battle, Bill's life transformed. He shed 35 pounds, regaining the best shape he'd been in since his high school days. Elijah had become more than just a colleague; he was an anchor, a source of inspiration and encouragement that breathed life into Bill's weary bones.

Their friendship extended beyond the walls of the hospital. They became like brothers, brothers in arms on the front lines of a war that raged on a different front, a front unseen by most. They fought with the conviction that their actions, like soldiers preventing nuclear catastrophe on a distant battlefield, could save the world from the dire consequences of a relentless virus.

Together, they learned to find strength in one another, to lean on the collective wisdom, resilience, and unspoken camaraderie that held them together. In the heart of the hellscape, they were bound by a shared mission, an unspoken oath to face the darkness head-on and emerge victorious. These brothers, forged in the crucible of the pandemic, were a testament to the strength of the human spirit when faced with insurmountable odds.

Brothers of the
Pandemic Frontline

In the heart of the battle,
they stood as one,
Brothers of the frontline,
under the relentless sun,
Their unwavering spirits,
never to be undone,
In the hellscape,
their stories had just begun.

Jermaine, the elder with wisdom to share,
In emergencies, his composure was rare,
With intubation skills, beyond compare,
A beacon of hope in healthcare's despair.

Elijah, the young, with strength that amazed,
Working endless shifts, his spirit unfazed,
To the gym he'd go, where strength blazed,
In the darkest hours, his dedication blazed.

Bill, who'd fought his own inner war,
Found a friend in Elijah,
who'd gone to the core,
Lost pounds, gained strength,
as their spirits soared,
Brothers in arms,
their bond they'd explore.

Their story,
a testament to resilience and grace,
In the hellscape, they found a sacred space,
Together they stood, a formidable embrace,
Brothers of the frontline,
in this challenging place.

Through the darkest hours,
they'd always strive,
For in unity and courage,
they'd truly come alive,
In the pandemic's fire,
they'd learn to survive,
Brothers of the frontline,
stories of heroes, they'd derive.

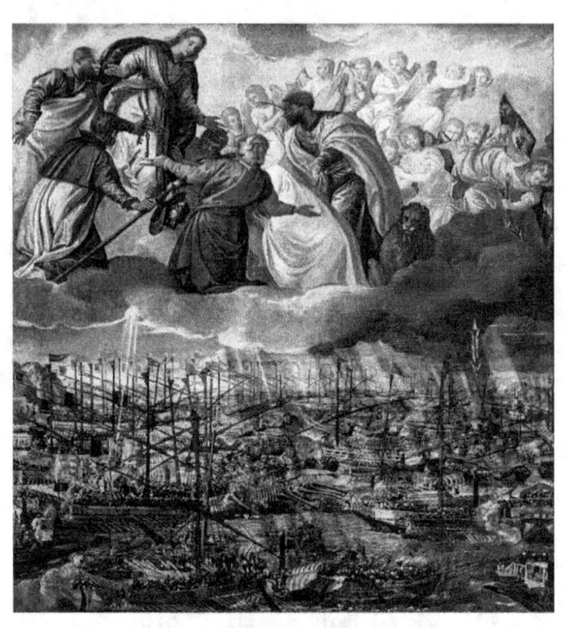

Revelation 6:9-11

When he opened the fifth seal, I saw underneath the altar the souls of those who had been killed for the Word of God, and for the testimony of the Christ which they had. [10] They cried with a loud voice, saying, "How long, Master, the holy and true, until you judge and avenge our blood on those evil lab scientists who released the Covid-19 virus on the earth?" [11] A long white robe was given to each of them. They were told that they should rest yet for a while, until their fellow servants and their brothers,[§] who would also be killed even as they were, should complete their course.*

**Modified a verse to reflect a nightmare Bill had after reading his Bible before going to bed.*

Chapter Nine

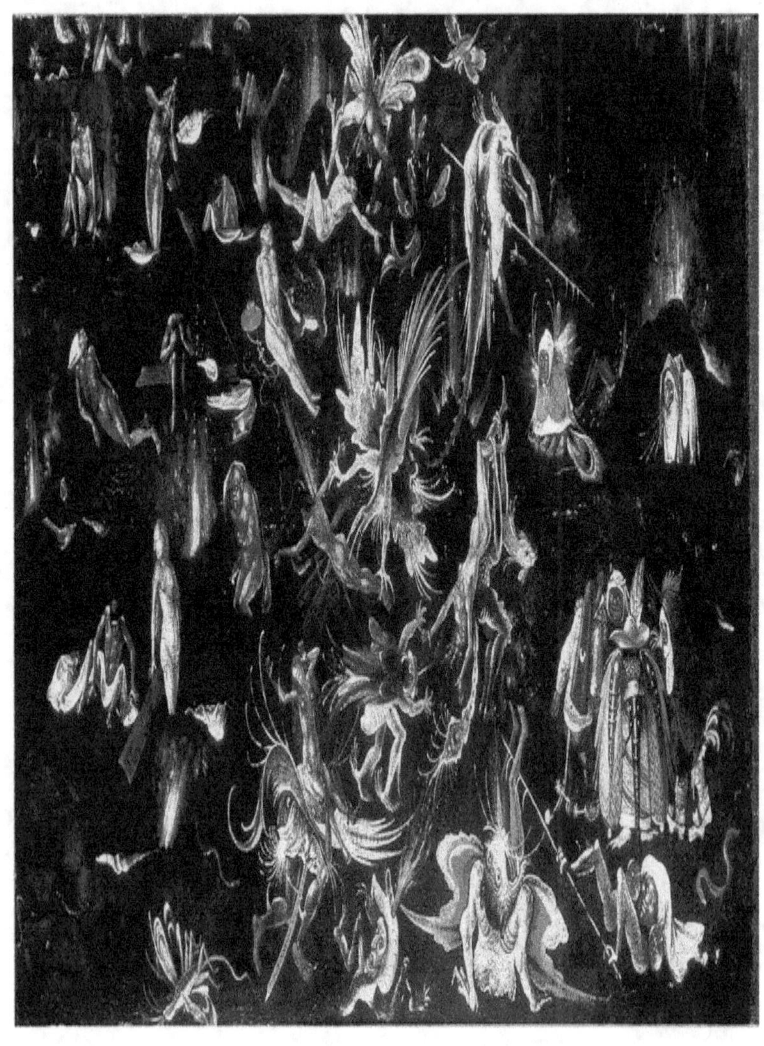

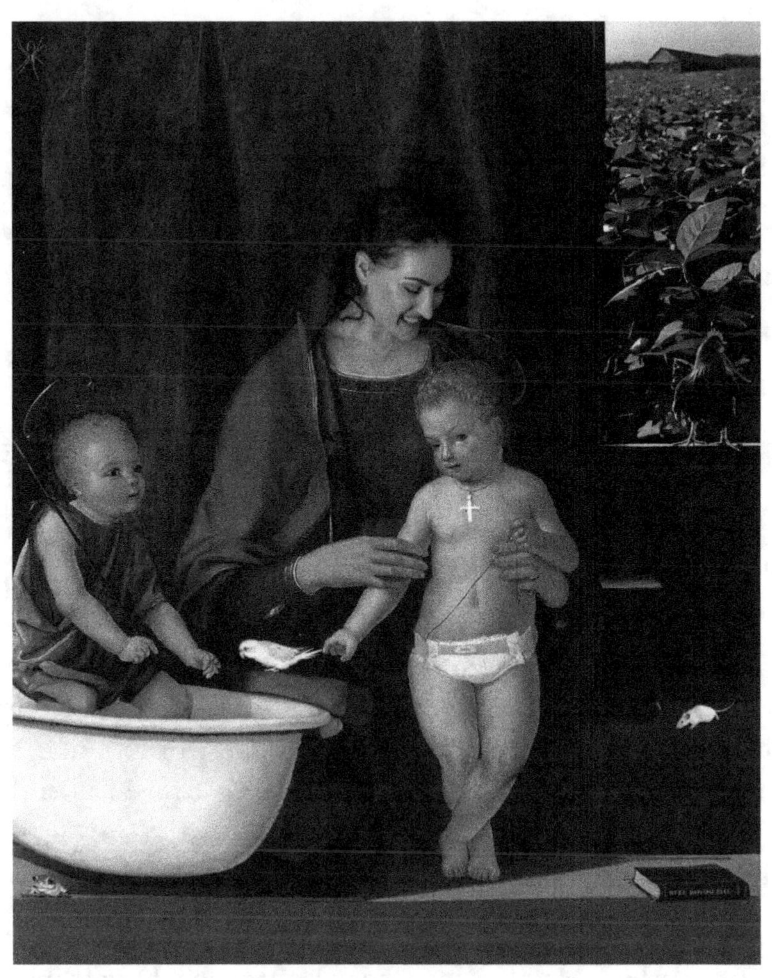

Proverbs 31:26-28

She opens her mouth with wisdom.
Kind instruction is on her tongue.
27 She looks well to the ways of her household,
and doesn't eat the bread of idleness.
28 Her children grow up and call her blessed.

Her Love and Wisdom

In the heart of the pandemic's relentless storm, Bill, the dedicated Respiratory Therapist, found himself facing a series of trials that would test his resilience and faith. Having been vaccinated three times prior to catching COVID-19, he was taken aback when the virus struck not once, but twice.

The first time he contracted the virus, even after receiving three FDA vaccinations prior, the battle was arduous. He fought the fever, cough, and fatigue, knowing that his role as a healthcare worker made him more susceptible. With courage and determination, he overcame the virus's grip, emerged on the other side, and returned to his mission of saving lives.

However, the pandemic continued to rage on, relentless and unyielding. The hospital corridors echoed with the struggles of countless patients, and the toll on healthcare workers like Bill was immeasurable. Day after day, he bore witness to over 300 patients losing their lives, the virus serving as the instigating factor that brought about their swift descent into the depths of death.

In the midst of this dark period, Bill received devastating news. His mother, Marilyn, had been courageously battling cancer for over a decade, a silent and relentless adversary of her own. As Bill saw the lives he could not save slip away, he faced the looming shadow of his mother's impending loss.

The day came when Marilyn, the woman who had been his rock and the source of his inspiration, passed away. Her absence left a void in Bill's heart, a profound sense of loss that could not be filled. Grief washed over him, and he felt as if the world had crumbled beneath his feet.

In the depths of his despair, Bill found solace in the memory of his mother's unwavering faith. She had been a source of inspiration throughout his life, her love and wisdom guiding him through every trial. It was her voice that echoed in his mind, reminding him to find strength in faith during the darkest hours. And to attend the assemblies of the Church of Christ for support that towers.

Bill turned to God, seeking solace and strength in his mother's memory. As he leaned on his faith, he discovered an unyielding resilience within himself, a determination to continue fighting the pandemic despite the darkness that surrounded him.

When the next wave of COVID-19 arrived, Bill faced it with a newfound sense of purpose. His faith had not only brought him closer to God but also closer to the depths of his own strength. He knew that his mother's spirit would always be with him, guiding him through the toughest times.

In the heart of the pandemic, Bill, a survivor of COVID-19 twice over, found his inspiration not only in the lives he saved but in the memory of the woman who had raised him to be a beacon of hope and compassion. In her memory, he vowed to carry on, knowing that his work in the hospital was not just a job, but a tribute to the unwavering love of a mother and a testament to the resilience of the human spirit.

Her Love and Wisdom

In the heart of the pandemic's darkest days,

Bill faced a path of challenging ways,

COVID struck him twice,

with a relentless blaze,

Yet, in his heart,

his mother's love always stays.

Vaccinated thrice, the battle was rough,

In his role,

where lives hung by a thread so tough,

With courage and faith, he would rebuff,

The virus's grip, when it seemed so gruff.

Through hospital corridors,

the struggle did roar,

Over 300 patients,

lost in the pandemic's war,

Their descent into darkness,

a pain to explore,

For Bill, each loss,

an ache to his core.

But in the midst of the pandemic's despair,

He received news,

a burden too heavy to bear,

His mother, Marilyn, had gone,

no longer there,

A loss so deep, a cross too hard to bear.

Her memory, a beacon,

in his heart, did gleam,

She'd inspired him to fight,

to fulfill his dream,

With her love and wisdom,

like a gentle stream,

Guiding him through the toughest pandemic scheme.

In her memory,

Bill turned to the divine,

A newfound faith,

where his spirit would shine,

He drew strength from the heavens' design,

For in his mother's love,

he'd intertwine.

The next COVID wave,

he faced with grace,

His mother's spirit,

a presence to embrace,

A testament to the human spirit's embrace,

A legacy of love,

in every single space.

In the heart of the pandemic's deepest strife,

Bill's journey, filled with courage and life,

For in his mother's memory,

amidst the strife,

He found the strength to carry on,

and thrive.

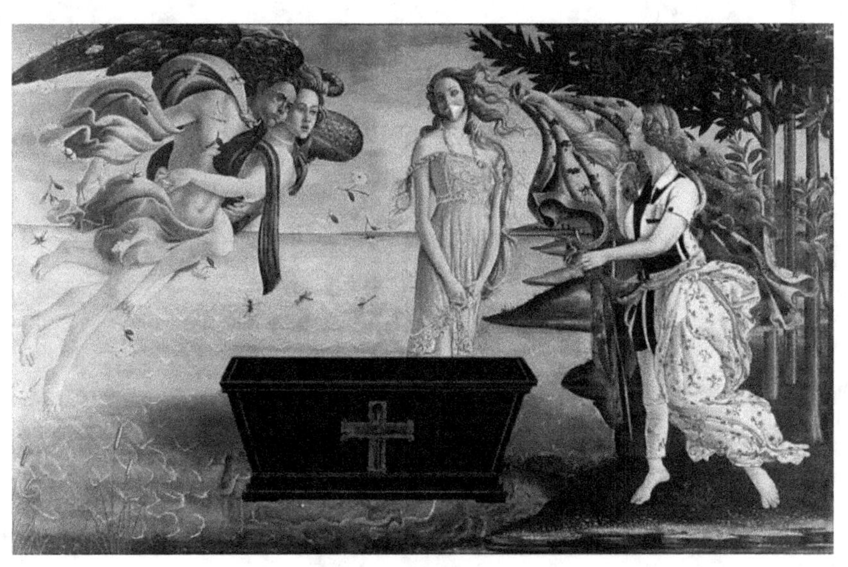

1 Thessalonians 4:13-18

But we don't want you to be uninformed, brothers and sisters, concerning those who have fallen asleep, so that you don't grieve like the rest, who have no hope. 14 For if we believe that Jesus died and rose again, even so God will bring with him those who have fallen asleep in Jesus. 15 For this we tell you by the word of the Lord, that we who are alive, who are left until the coming of the Lord, will in no way precede those who have fallen asleep. 16 For the Lord himself will descend from heaven with a shout, with the voice of the archangel and with God's trumpet. The dead in Christ will rise first, 17 then we who are alive, who are left, will be caught up together with them in the clouds to meet the Lord in the air. So we will be with the Lord forever. 18 Therefore comfort one another with these words.

Chapter Ten

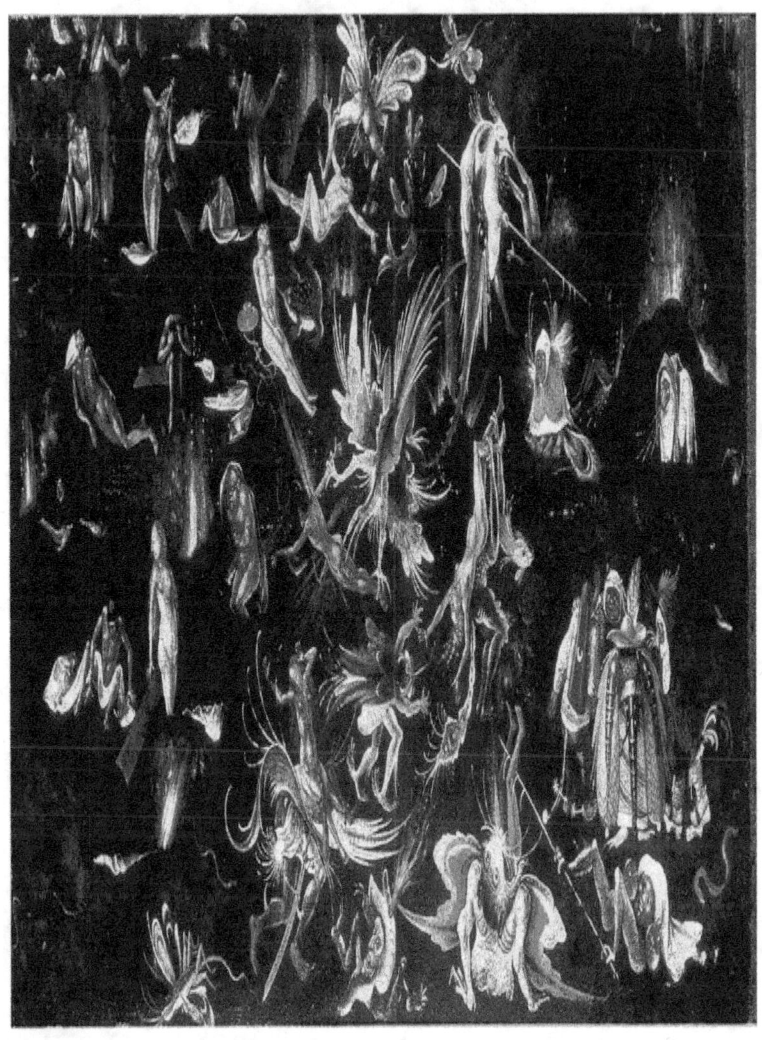

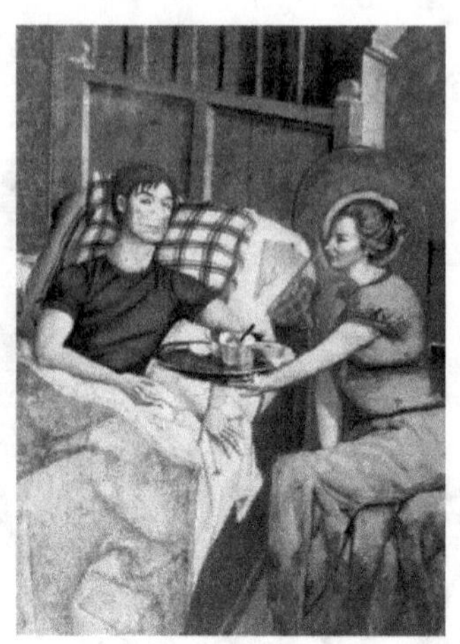

Proverbs 31:10-12

A man should search for a worthy woman to marry. For her value is far above precious jewels.[11] *The heart of her husband trusts in her. He shall have no lack of gain.*[12] *She does him good, and not harm, all the days of her life.*

In the Arms of Love

As the sun dipped below the horizon, casting a warm, orange glow over the quiet neighborhood, Bill sat in his favorite armchair, feeling exhausted and defeated. The past few weeks had been a relentless battle, and he had been on the losing side, facing an invisible enemy: COVID-19. His strength had dwindled, and even the simplest tasks now felt like insurmountable mountains. The once-vigorous Respiratory Therapist had become a patient, relying on the care of his wonderful and compassionate wife, Andrea.

It had all started when Bill developed a persistent cough, and his body began to ache as if a thousand tiny arrows had pierced his muscles. When the results of the COVID-19 test came back positive, he knew he was in for a rough ride. Isolation became his new reality, and the loneliness weighed heavily on his spirit.

Andrea, a woman of boundless empathy and love, had always been his pillar of support. Now, she took on the role of caregiver with unwavering dedication. Every morning, she put on a mask, gown, and gloves, just as Bill had done countless times before, to bring him breakfast and medicine. But her true strength lay in her soothing presence. She sat beside him, holding his hand and speaking words of encouragement as if her voice had the power to chase away the virus itself.

"You're going to get through this, Bill," she would say, her eyes filled with determination. "We'll beat this together."

Bill's symptoms worsened, and there were nights when he felt like he couldn't breathe, when the walls of their bedroom seemed to close in on him. In those moments, Andrea became his lifeline. She would help him sit up, propping him with pillows, and she'd stay by his side through the long, fearful nights.

One particularly difficult night, Bill's fever soared. He was drenched in sweat, his body trembling uncontrollably. Andrea, her voice trembling with worry, called the hospital for advice. The doctor on the other end of the line reassured her and provided guidance on how to manage the fever.

Andrea soaked a cloth in cool water and gently placed it on Bill's forehead. She spoke to him in soft, soothing tones, sharing stories of their happiest moments together, as if their cherished memories could chase away the illness.

Weeks passed, and Bill's condition began to improve, albeit slowly. His coughing fits became less frequent, and his energy levels showed signs of returning. Andrea's tireless care and unwavering love had undoubtedly played a pivotal role in his recovery.

One sunny morning, as Bill sat in the armchair by the window, he looked out at the world with fresh eyes. The vibrant colors of the garden and the cheerful chirping of birds were like a balm to his soul. He turned to Andrea, his eyes filled with gratitude and love.

"Andrea, you're my rock," he whispered, his voice weak but filled with sincerity. "I couldn't have done this without you."

Andrea's eyes glistened with tears, and she smiled warmly. "We've always been a team, Bill. In sickness and in health, remember? We're in this together."

As Bill continued to regain his strength, he knew that the road to a full recovery would still be long and challenging. But with Andrea by his side, with her compassion, unwavering support, and love, he found the hope and determination to face whatever lay ahead.

Together, they had navigated the storm of his illness, and their love had emerged even stronger, a testament to the power of their unbreakable bond.

In the Arms of Love

In the Arms of Love,
where Bill lay,
Battling the tempest,
a challenging day,
With COVID's grip,
in his humble abode,
He found strength in Andrea,
their love bestowed.

Through fevered nights
and the weakest of hours,
Andrea's compassion was
a garden of flowers,
She tended to him,
with unwavering grace,
A guardian angel,
in that sacred space.

In the cocoon of home,
where recovery began,
Andrea's love was a healing,
a miraculous plan,
She soothed his fears,
brought warmth to the cold,
Their love's fire burned bright,
a story to be told.

In the arms of love, Bill found his way,
From darkness to dawn, in the struggle's ballet,
Andrea, the compass, in the journey they wove,
Their love, the anthem, of resilience and trove.

Through the battles they faced, together they'd strive,
In the arms of love, their spirits alive,
A tale of courage, in the darkness they'd see,
Andrea and Bill, where love's victory will be.

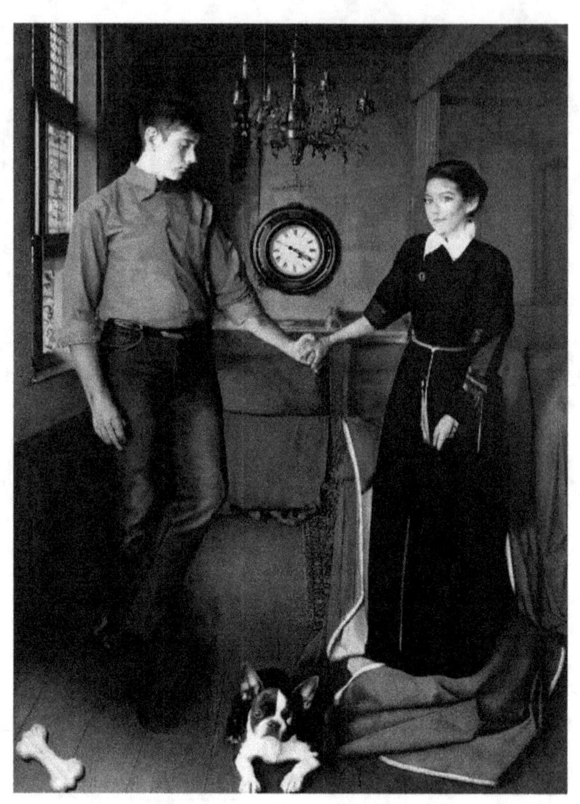

Ephesians 5:25-28

Husbands, love your wives, even as Christ also loved the church and gave himself up for them, 26 that he might sanctify them, having cleansed them by the washing of water with the word, 27 that he might present the church to God gloriously, not having spot or wrinkle, but that they should be holy and without defect. 28 Even so husbands also ought to love their own wives as their own bodies. He who loves his own wife loves himself.

Chapter Eleven

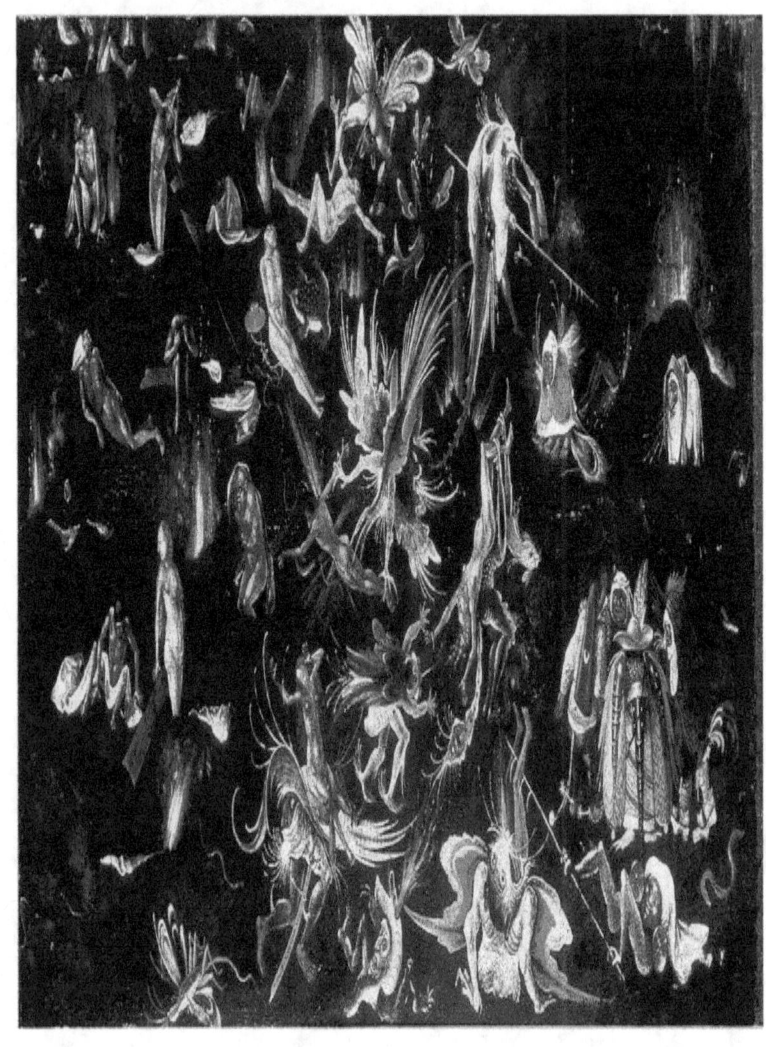

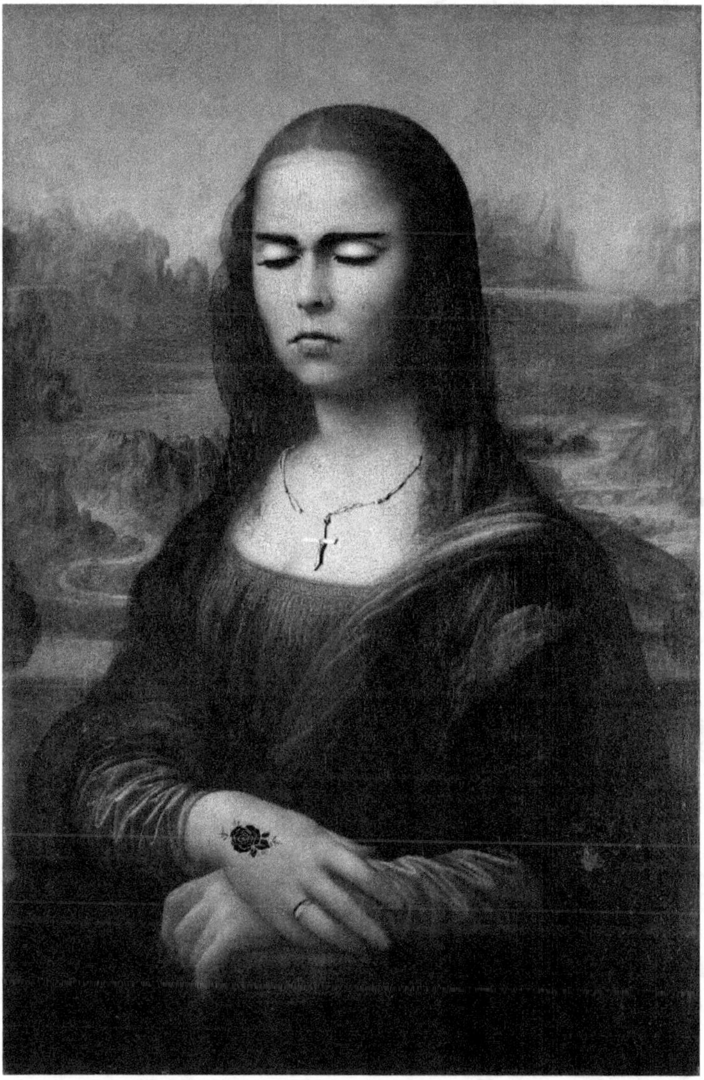

John 15:13

**Greater love has no one than this,
that someone lay down their life
for their friends.**

Maria's Eternal Light

Bill's journey through the depths of the COVID-19 pandemic had been one of resilience and recovery. Having battled the virus twice, with the unwavering support of his compassionate wife, Andrea, he had emerged from the shadows, stronger and more determined than ever. When he finally returned to work at the hospital, it was with a renewed sense of purpose and a deep appreciation for life.

The hospital was not the same place he had left. The relentless waves of the virus had taken a heavy toll, and the loss of colleagues and friends weighed on everyone's hearts. But Bill was determined to carry on, to be a beacon of hope for his patients and a source of strength for his remaining coworkers.

It was a bright, sunny morning when he arrived at the hospital, with his PPE in place and a sense of optimism in his heart. As he walked through the familiar corridors, the memories of the battles fought here, and the lives saved, filled him with a mix of emotions. He couldn't help but smile as he thought about the tremendous sacrifices and the victories they had achieved.

However, as he entered the ICU, the atmosphere was somber. The news of Maria's passing had spread like wildfire. She, the spirited nurse who had been a ray of sunshine in the darkest of days, had succumbed to the very enemy they had fought so valiantly against.

The ICU, once filled with the bustle of healthcare workers, was now a place of mourning. Colleagues huddled together, tears glistening in their eyes, sharing stories of Maria's kindness, her laughter, and her unwavering dedication to her patients. Her absence was a void that could never be filled.

Bill stood there, a heavy heart, and tears welled up in his eyes. He remembered Maria's warmth, her smile that could light up even the gloomiest of days. She had been his companion through some of the toughest times, and now she was gone.

In that moment, he made a silent promise. He would carry on Maria's legacy, ensuring that her compassion and dedication would live on in the care he provided. As he cared for the patients, he whispered words of comfort and hope, just as Maria had done. Her memory fueled his determination to save lives and to provide solace in the face of despair.

In the days that followed, Bill worked tirelessly, reminded of the fragility of life and the importance of every moment. Maria's spirit was with him, guiding him through the darkest of hours. He shared her stories with new colleagues, ensuring that her memory would continue to inspire others.

Maria's passing was a stark reminder of the sacrifices made by countless healthcare workers, the heroes who stood at the forefront of the pandemic. It was a painful chapter in their journey, but one that only reinforced their commitment to saving lives and honoring the memories of those they had lost.

In the midst of grief and loss, Bill, the survivor of COVID-19, the husband of a supportive wife, and the friend of many, continued to stand strong. He knew that in the face of adversity, the human spirit could shine its brightest, and that even in the depths of sorrow, there was room for hope and inspiration.

Maria's Eternal Light

In the quiet of the hospital's halls,
A solemn echo of life's calls,
Bill returned, a hero of yore,
To a battlefield where angels soar.

Among the heroes, he sought to find,
Maria, a friend of heart and mind,
But the news he heard was a shattering gale,
For Maria's light, the world did assail.

A soul so bright, in the pandemic's grasp,
She fought with courage in each clasp,
But the relentless virus claimed its prey,
And Bill's heart wept on that fateful day.

Their bond was forged 'mid chaos and fear,
In the hospital's depths, ever near,
Now Maria's spirit takes its flight,
Beyond the stars, in eternal light.

In the heart of the hallowed space,
Bill held a memory's embrace,
Maria's legacy, in every case,
A poem of courage, a journey to trace.

For heroes like Bill, the fight goes on,
Though Maria's presence is forever gone,
In the halls of the hospital, they'll always dawn,
A tale of strength, though the tears may spawn.

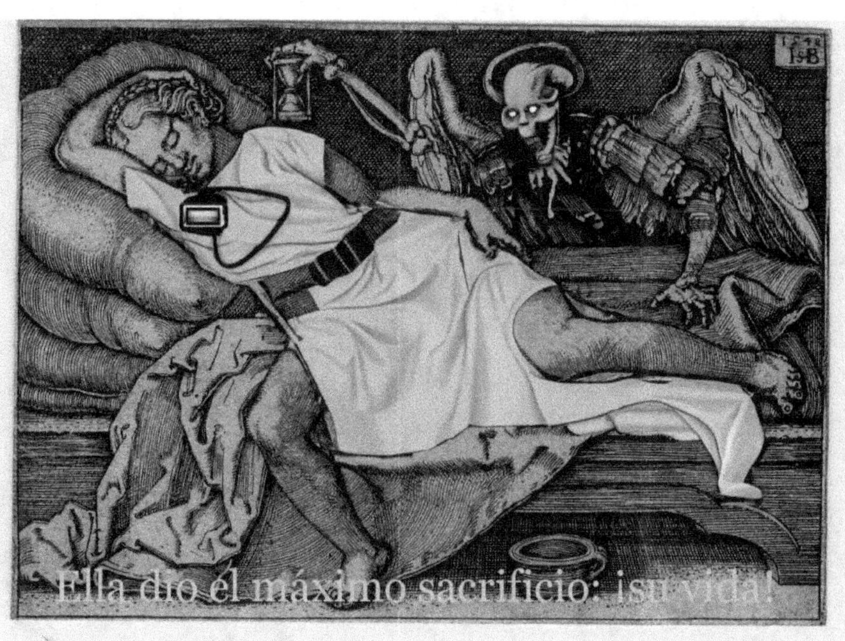

Matthew 10:28

*Don't be afraid of those who kill the body,
but are not able to kill the soul...*

Matthew 5:12

*Rejoice, and be exceedingly glad,
for great is your reward in heaven...*

Chapter Twelve

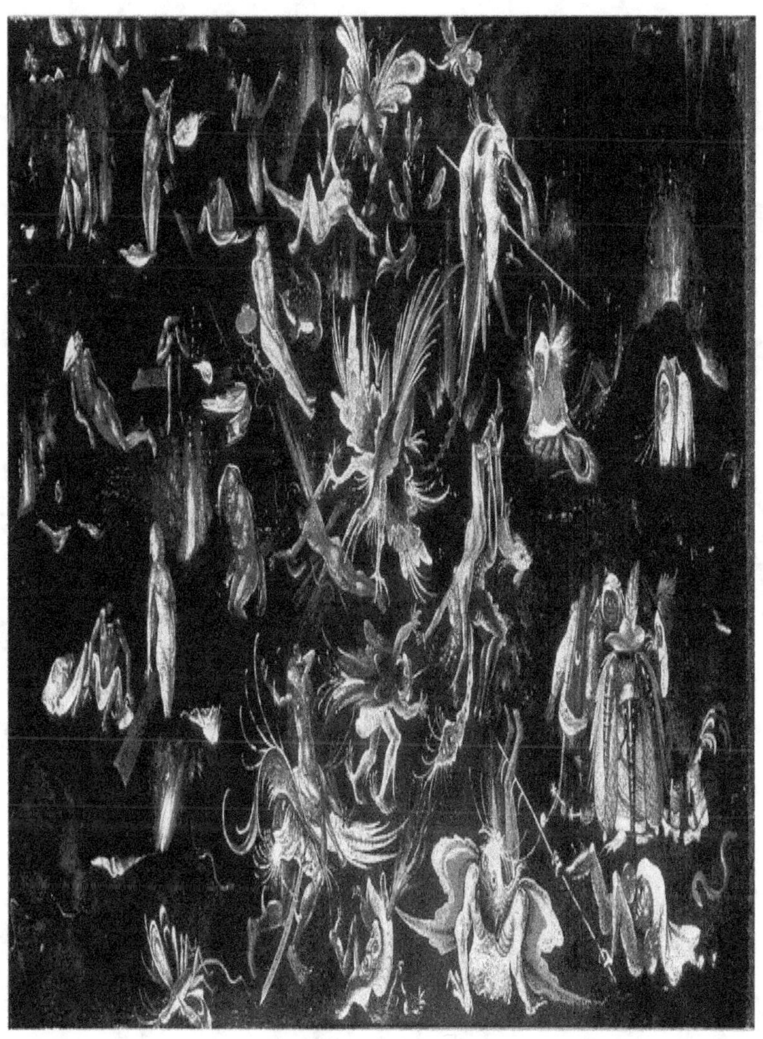

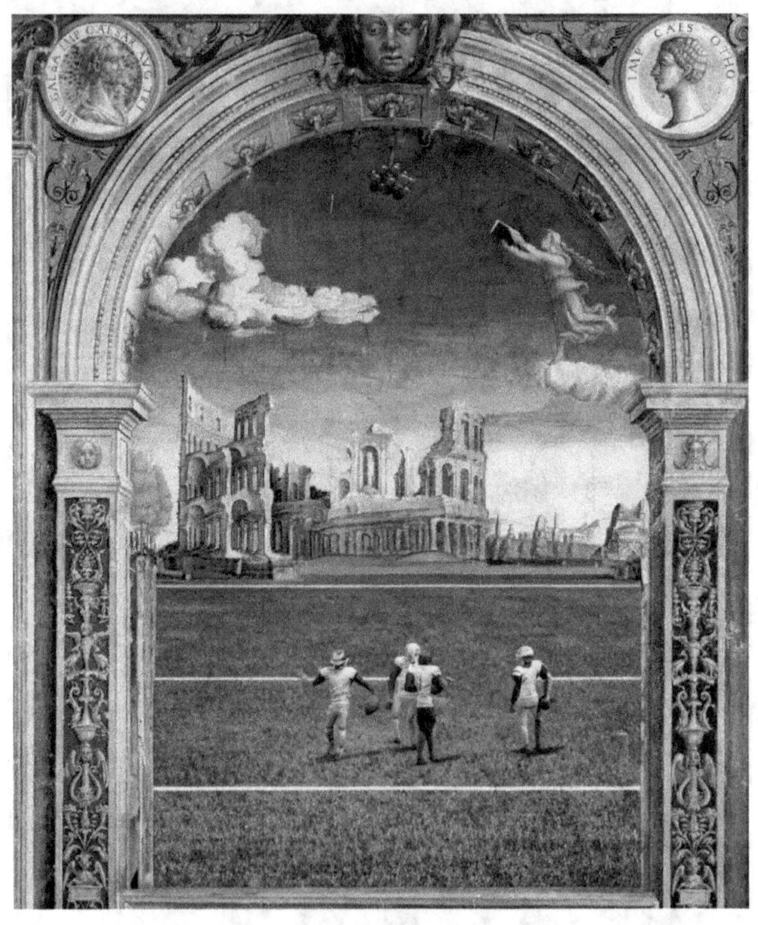

Philippians 4:13

*I can do all things
through Christ
who strengthens me.*

Our Coach's Resilience

Olivia McKinley had spent years working as a Respiratory Therapist, navigating the intricate dance of breath and life in the intensive care unit (ICU). Her experience had taught her to remain calm in the face of adversity, but nothing could have prepared her for the challenges that awaited her on a fateful day in the ICU.

Ron Pakora, a 47-year-old college men's football coach from Old South College in Rome, Georgia, had been admitted with severe double pneumonia due to Covid-19. The once robust and energetic coach was now fighting for every breath. As Olivia evaluated the vitals monitor, she could see the gravity of the situation in the lines and numbers on the screen.

Days turned into nights as Olivia tirelessly worked to stabilize Mr. Pakora's deteriorating condition. The ICU became a battleground, with the BiPAP pressure ventilating machine the only lifeline keeping the coach connected to the world. The hospital staff, aware of Mr. Pakora's significance to Old South College and the football community, rallied behind him, offering support and encouragement.

Then came the dreaded moment when Mr. Pakora went into respiratory failure, his body threatening to succumb to the merciless grip of the virus. Olivia, a seasoned professional, acted swiftly. In the chaos of a Code Blue, she skillfully intubated Mr. Pakora, securing a passage for life-saving breaths. Simultaneously, a dose of amiodarone coursed through the coach's veins, stabilizing his erratic heartbeat.

The ICU staff, with Olivia at the forefront, battled through the night, refusing to yield to the invisible enemy that had taken hold of Mr. Pakora's body. Flowers, cookies, and letters of encouragement poured in from fans, colleagues, and students, creating a small haven of hope amid the sterile hospital environment.

Weeks passed, and the ventilator became both a friend and a foe. It sustained Mr. Pakora's life, yet it also held him captive. Olivia's determination never wavered as she carefully monitored and adjusted the ventilator settings, waiting for the opportune moment to liberate the coach from its mechanical embrace.

Finally, after three long weeks, the day arrived when Olivia could begin the delicate process of weaning Mr. Pakora off the ventilator. It was a gradual journey, marked by small victories and setbacks. Yet, with each passing day, the coach's strength and resilience became evident. The ICU staff, fueled by the outpouring of support from the Old South community, witnessed a remarkable recovery.

Two weeks later, Mr. Pakora, with a weak but genuine smile, walked out of the ICU, leaving behind a room that had been both a battlefield and a sanctuary. The cheers from the Old South fans echoed in the corridors as he reunited with his family, grateful for the second chance at life.

A year later, Old South College hosted a grand pep rally to celebrate the resilience of their beloved coach and to express gratitude to the healthcare heroes who had played a pivotal role in his recovery. Mr. Pakora, now back in the vibrant world of football, took the stage with humility and gratitude.

In a heartfelt moment, he welcomed Olivia McKinley to the assembly, acknowledging the Respiratory Therapist's crucial role in his journey back to health. The applause was thunderous as Olivia, a modest hero in her own right, stood before the crowd, grateful for the opportunity to witness the power of perseverance and the unwavering support of a community that extended beyond the football field.

Our Coach's Resilience

In the hallowed halls where whispers cease,
A tale of courage found its lease.
A coach, once strong, in shadows lay,
A respiratory dance, life's price to pay.

Olivia McKinley, the weaver of breath and grace,
Navigating storms in the ICU's embrace.
Double pneumonia's cruel hand,
Yet hope persisted, a resilient stand.

Old South's coach, Ron Pakora, lay,
In the grip of illness, a fierce dismay.
Ventilator whispers, a lifeline thin,
As prayers and cheers converged within.

Code Blue echoed, a dire refrain,
Olivia's skilled hands, breaking illness' chain.
Intubation's dance, a desperate plea,
Amiodarone's rhythm, a symphony.

Flowers, cookies, letters of light,
From fans and kin, a beacon bright.
In the sterile realm, a community's plea,
A coach's battle against the unseen enemy.

Weeks passed, in the ICU's domain,
Ventilator's hold, a relentless strain.
Olivia, a guardian in the quiet night,
Fighting shadows, kindling hope's light.

With patience and skill, a slow release,
Weaning breath, the promise of peace.
Old South's cheers, a distant song,
As coach and therapist proved the strong.

A journey marked by victories small,
Resilience echoed in the hospital hall.
Released from the grip of cold despair,
Ron Pakora, in the open air.

A year unfurls, a grand rally's call,
Old South's pride, resilient and tall.
Coach Pakora, a beacon in the night,
Olivia McKinley, a silent hero, in healing's light.

" Our Coach's Resilience" the tale we sing,
Of courage, hope, and a respiratory wing.
In the dance of breath, life's symphony,
A coach reborn, a hero's legacy.

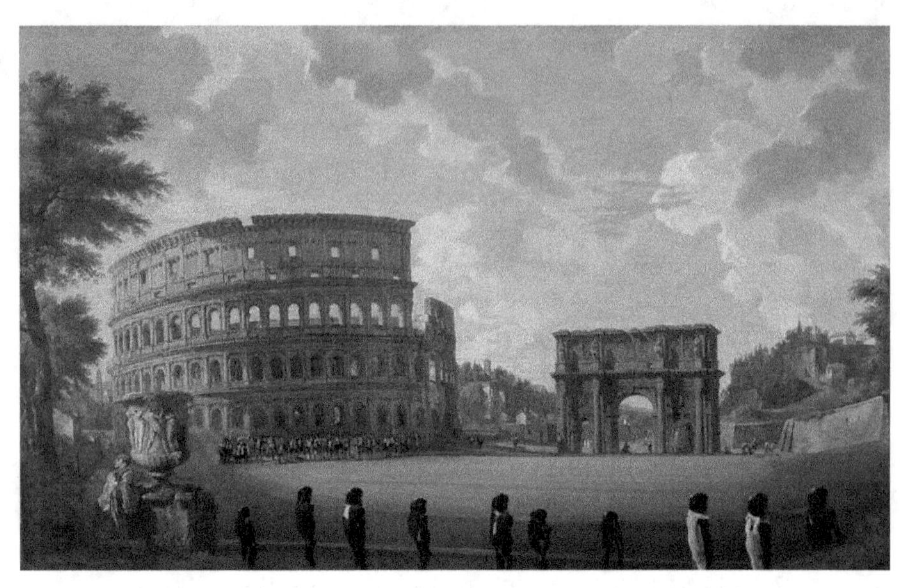

Hebrews 10:24-25

*Let's consider how to
influence one another
to love and perform good works,
not forgetting our own
assembling together,
as the custom of some is,
but encouraging one another,
and so much the more
as you see the Day approaching.*

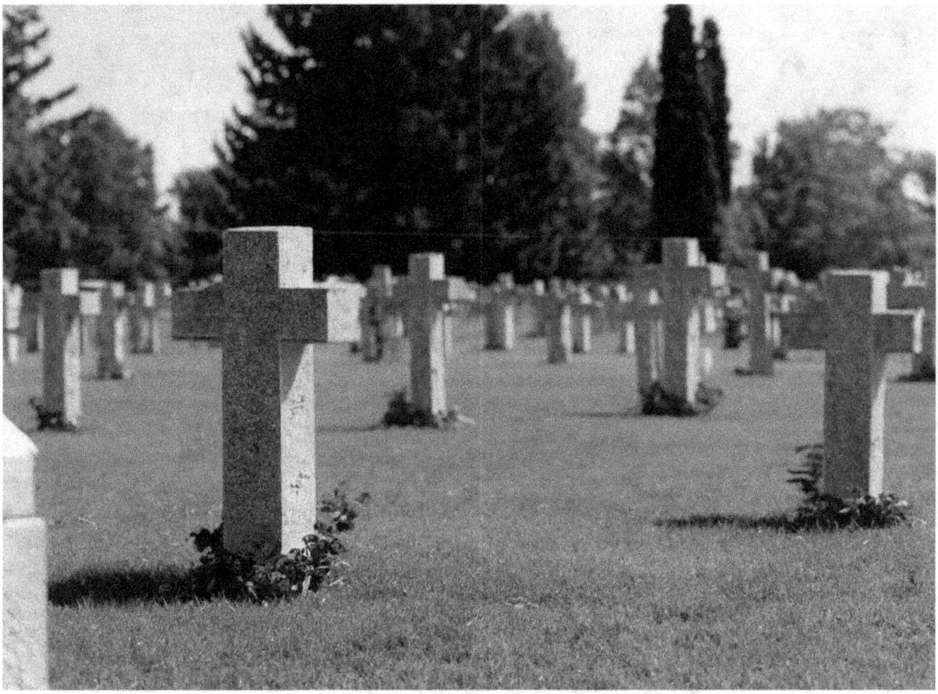

In Memoriam

To all the healthcare workers worldwide

Who sacrificed their lives on the frontlines

Of the Covid-19 Pandemic.

May God rest their souls

For dying as heroes.

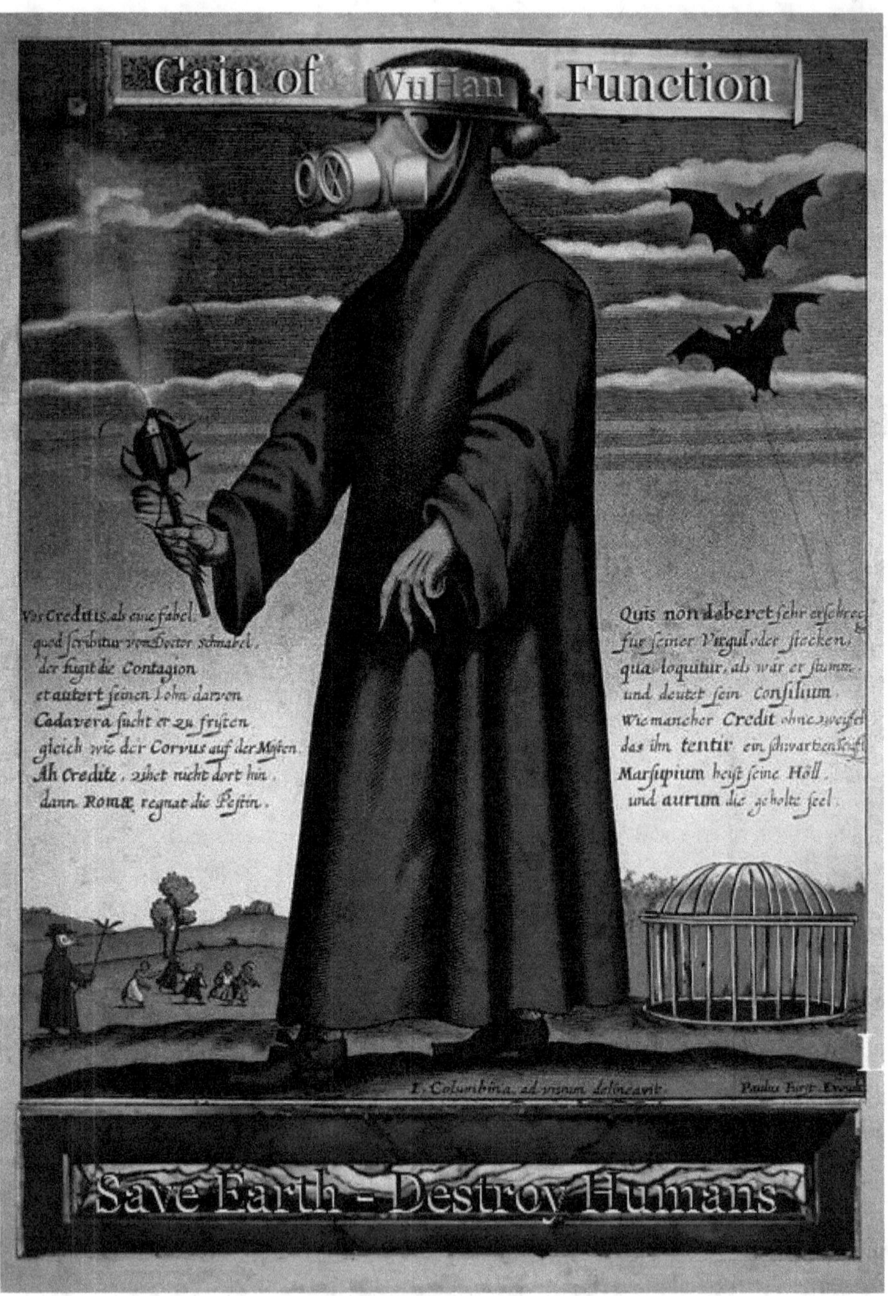

Gain of WuHan Function

Vos Creditis als eine fabel
quod scribitur von Doctor schnabel
der fugit die Contagion
et aufert seinen Lohn darvon
Cadavera sucht er zu frÿsten
gleich wie der Corvus auf der Mÿsten
Ah Credite, sihet nicht dort hin
dann ROMÆ regnat die Pestin.

Quis non deberet sehr erschrec
fur seiner Virgul oder stecken
quia loquitur, als wär er stumm
und deutet sein Consilium
Wie mancher Credit ohne zweyfel
das ihn tentir ein schwartzen keÿf
Marsupium heyst seine Höll
und aurum die geholte seel.

I. Columbina ad vivum delineavit.   Paulus Furst Excud.

Save Earth - Destroy Humans

The End

www.ingramcontent.com/pod-product-compliance
Lightning Source LLC
Chambersburg PA
CBHW070812260726

48660CB00005B/1820